Bangladeshi Fishes
Nutritions
Guide

I0124506

MAYAR AKASH

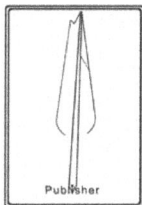

MA PUBLISHER

Waiver

Please note that the information in this book has been collated over a period of time of 10 years and various research information as well as on-line sites. Please do not use this information as advice, it is only for information to base or start from; you need to do your own due diligence or compare with source other than what is in this book.

The author and the publisher do not and will not accept responsibility for person using this information as advice. While the original research started back in 2014, and a basic guide was published with pictures and names, eversince then I have been researching to put togethered researched information about the nutritions of the Bangladeshi fishes. So fast forward to 2024, where I have finaly found ease with ChatGPT 3.5 & 4.0. With this I have been able to polish this version up with the generic information I was putting together, just as a "step onto", to get our heads around reading and gauging the fishes that we eat, which are not indiginness and aremainly imported in.

How to use the book

Use the book to identify the fish that you eat, want to eat or finding out about before you eat. The book is design to give you an overview of what they are and what they have. So if you want to know what you have been eating, this will give you an over view. If you want to know which fish is more benefitial, then you will get an overview of which fish is more nutritious. We have organised the information/data in a variety of ways for readers.

3

Acknowledgements

I would like show acknowledgement and gratitude to the following photographers who made this book possible to put together. They have remotely been doing their bit by taking photos of the small and various fishes in Asian and around the world. They have uploaded the fish pictures to various websites such as fishbase and others.

The photographers are in no particular order:
- Khan, Mohammad Moazzam (FB)
- Biswas, Benoy Krishna
- Alam, Murshedul
- Balaram Mahalder (FB)
- Hamid Badar Osmany (FB)
- Al-Mamun, Md. Abdullah
- Randall, John E
- Shirantha, Ramani
- Bakalial, Bikramaditya
- Freitas, Rui
- Hasan, Mohammad Eusuf
- Small, Fred
- Rahman, A. K. A
- Roberts, Tyson R
- Åhlander, Erik
- Flescher, Don
- Mya Than Tun
- Gloerfelt-Tarp, Thomas

I would like to give thanks to websites such as the fishbase and BEfish who have a wide range of fishes listed and have been instrumental in forming this book.

CONTENT

Waiver	3
How To Use The Book	3
Acknowledgements	4
Introduction	9
Ayre	13
Bag Mass, Tiger Fish, Bagarius Family,	15
Bag Mass	16
Bang Mass (Goonch)	18
Bagna	20
Bashpata	22
Bassa	24
Batashi	26
Battum	28
Bele	30
Bime	32
Bream	34
Buwal	36
Carp (Common)	38
Carp (Mahseer)	40
Chandoo	42
Chapila	44
Chelapata	46
Chiring	48
Chitol	50
Chokko Bata	52
Churi/Cutlassfish	54
Darkina	56
Foli	58
Fresh Water Galda	60
Gawra	62
Gonia	64
Gozar	66
Harina	68
Herring	70
Hichiri Moila	72
Hilsha	74
Kakila	76
Kali Bawsh	78
Kalisha	80
Katla	82
Keski (Anchovy (Devil)	84
Keski (Anchovy (Spotty-Face)	86

Keski	88
Koi	90
Koral	92
Lohita/Loyta	94
Mackerel (Atlantic)	96
Mackerel (Indian)	98
Magur	100
Meni	102
Mocca	104
Mola	106
Mrigel	108
Nola	109
Mussel	110
Oyster	112
Pabda	114
Pangush	116
Pilchard	118
Pomfret Black	120
Prawn Indian	122
Prawns, Tiger Prawn Indian	124
Puti (Ticto)	126
Puti	128
Puti, Shor	130
Rani	132
Rita	134
Rohu	136
Salmon, Atlantic	138
Sardine	140
Shilong	142
Shing	144
Shoil	146
Shor Puti (Sarana)	148
Silver Belly	150
Snow Trout	152
Star Baim	154
Tailla	156
Taki	158
Tengra	160
Tengra (Striped)	162
Tengra, Gulsha	164
Tilapia	166
Trout (Rainbow)	168
Tuna (Skipjack)	170
Tuna (Yellowfin)	172

Essential Amino Acids And Their Health Benefits 174
Non-Essential Amino Acids And Their Health Benefits 175
Health Conditions Remedied By Specific Amino Acids 176
Non-Essential Amino Acids And Health Conditions 177
Health Conditions Remedied By Minerals Found In Fish 178
Can You Have Too Much Fish? 180
Summary And Recommendations 181
Best Ways To Prepare And Eat Fish For Maximum Health Benefits 182
Additional Tips For Healthy Fish Consumption 183
Oiliest Fish Known To Man 184
Atlantic Mackerel (Scomber Scombrus) 184
Other Notably Oily Fish 184
Consumption Recommendations 185
Bangladeshi Fish And Diabetes 185
Specific Benefits For Managing Diabetes 186
Practical Tips For Incorporating Fish Into A Diabetic Diet 186
1. Salmon (Salmo Salar) 187
2. Mackerel (Scomber Scombrus) 187
3. Sardines (Sardinella Spp.) 187
4. Trout (Oncorhynchus Mykiss) 187
5. Herring (Clupea Harengus) 187
6. Tuna (Thunnus Spp.) 188
Mechanisms Of Anti-Diabetic Effects 188
Additional Recommendations 188
Bangladeshi Fish And Psoriasis 189
1. Hilsa (Tenualosa Ilisha) 189
2. Rohu (Labeo Rohita) 189
3. Catla (Catla Catla) 189
4. Tilapia (Oreochromis Niloticus) 189
5. Pangasius (Pangasius Pangasius) 189
Specific Benefits For Managing Psoriasis 189
Practical Tips For Incorporating Fish Into A Psoriasis-Friendly Diet 190
Anti-Aging And Fish 190
1. Salmon (Salmo Salar) 190
2. Hilsa (Tenualosa Ilisha) 190
3. Mackerel (Scomber Scombrus) 190
4. Rohu (Labeo Rohita) 191
5. Catla (Catla Catla) 191
6. Sardines (Sardinella Longiceps) 191
7. Tuna (Thunnus Spp.) 191
8. Tilapia (Oreochromis Niloticus) 191
Nutritional Components Beneficial For Anti-Aging 191
Practical Tips 191
Blood Group Compatibility With Bangladeshi Fish 191

7

Bangladeshi Fish With Low Glycemic Index   192
   Bangladeshi Fish That May Help Prevent Heart Attacks   192
Here Are Some Bangladeshi Fish Known To Be Beneficial For Heart Health: 192
Immune Booster Fishes   193
   Additional Recommendations   194
Fish Combinations To Avoid   194
   General Tips   194
Mercury   195
Effects Of Mercury Consumption Through Fish   195
Mercury Levels In Fish By Region   196
   General Trends   196
Types Of Mercury Found In Fish By Region   196
   Regional Highlights   197
   Conclusion   197
References/ Sources   198
   Example References   199

Introduction

As a Bangladeshi growing up in the United Kingdom, I did not get this education about the fishes of Bangladesh and ones that we consume on a daily basis. If I was in Bangladeshi, purchasing fish would have been a daily occurrence and also having links to the village I would have gone fishing. I did have a go when I was in Bangladesh (1984), young and I went into the paddy fields to catch small fishes in my cords trousers rolled up to my knees and bare footed into the clay mud, with thorns, twigs and lillypads. That was short lived but the experience lifes on with me as if it happened yesterday.

In UK, many like me who have grown up in UK have very limited knowledge about the fishes. It is very daunting and embarrassing to go to the Asian grocery shops and ask what they are. It was ok when I was younger but now that I am older near to half a century its different, a part of knowledge and identity is missing, as your surrender that the very moment you ask the question.

It has taken me over a decade to slowly at a snails pace to put this book together, the actual research and sources were very specific and more to the point, research papers that needed and scientist brain to decifer the results. With the research, I was in the hands of the researcher, who did their own peer revue papers, and there would be small sample or specific aspects covered and not what the information that I was working towards. I did put together the information but run into dead ends, so a little while ago, I decided to publish a pictoral book with the Bangladeshi fishes with tables in to use it as a fish identifier and to make obervastional recordings, and it fell sort of what I wanted to achieve, and what individuals had said to me, in regards to having a book that give the nutritional informations, such as fat content, vitamisn, minerals and amino cids content of the fishes.

Since that basic book publication, I perserviered with the research and have been trowling through the research paperwork and collating the figures. Getting the full spectrum of the nutritional information was same as where you catch many of the fishes from, an "Ocean", the web was the ocean of information, and I was slowly making progress.

So, early on I desisted to use the ChatGPT 2.0, which I did use for another subject, and I also did try and asked the questions about the fish and the nutrition, it had no information; and that is where that stayed. So, recently in a random conversation with a family member, who had some joy in using the newer version of Chatgpt3.5, and that triggered me to test it again, to see if it has any information about my research.

To my surprise, ChatGpt 4.0 had information about the information I was seeking, but then again I uploaded the whole document, and found that it was extracting information from that. I then got sceptical, so I started a new thread, chat, and it started finding information that I was looking for. This was a sigh of relief, it was finding the information I was telling it to.

At that point, the feeling I experienced was of, as if I had put a "1000 horse powered engine to a mule pulling a cart up the mountain side". I have achieved to put together with the assistance of chatgpt3.5/4.0 in matter of weeks, then what I have achieved in a decade. The stats are average from the source, as listed at the back of the book.

This also helped me put together a list of questions that I wanted information to as I have been researching for personal reasons. I have been looking into psoriasis, heart disease, diabetes and cholesterol. I have know been ables to put together a list of benefitial fishes.

So this book is to help all and anyone who wants to have a guide to assist them is knowing and selecting fishes when they go to the fish mongers.

84 sea fishes, shell fish and molluscs covered in this book, you have them now clearly listed in the following order:

1. Fish name, common and scientific, with picture – to identify
2. Oil content
3. Omegas
4. Cholestrol level
5. Sodium level
6. Mercury level
7. Nutritional information
   a. Calories
   b. Proteins
   c. Fat
8. Vitamins
9. Minerals
10. Amino Acids
11. Essential Amino Acids And Their Health Benefits
12. Health Conditions Remedied By Minerals Found In Fish
13. Bangladeshi Fish And Diabetes
14. Bangladeshi Fish And Psoriasis
15. Anti-Aging And Fish
16. Blood Group Compatibility With Bangladeshi Fish
17. Bangladeshi Fish With Low Glycemic Index
18. Effects Of Mercury Consumption Through Fish

All this information was my long term research goal and I was able to achieve a mile stone, an understanding of the common knowledge and fish and how they support us. So, all of you, this is a generic information, to facilitate learning and further research and studies to pin point the knowledge of our well being and fish. Please use this as general information, and **not** as medical fact or guidance, use this to get a starting point for your own detective work.

It has taken over a decade to get it to this stage; I hope this brings some order, comfort and joy in knowing the fishes you eat, and this include non Bangladeshi fishes too.

FISHES & NUTRITION

Ayre

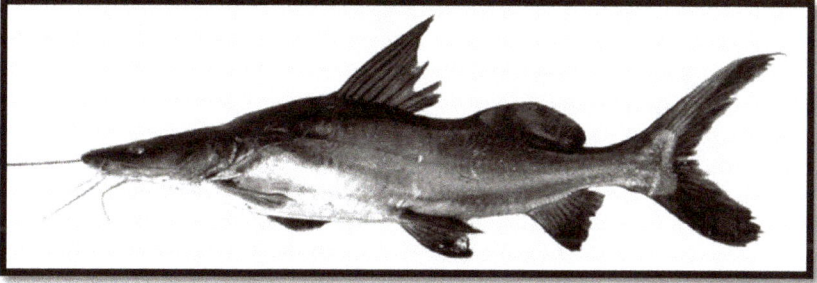

Nutritional Profile of Mystus Aor

Common Name: Ayre   **Scientific Name**: Mystus /Sperata Aor

1. Oil Content
- **Category**: Medium
- **Oil Breakdown**: Contains a balance of healthy fats, including omega-3 and omega-6 fatty acids.

2. Omega Fatty Acids
- **Omega-3**: Moderate
- **Omega-6**: Present
- **Omega-9**: Minor amounts

3. Cholesterol Content
- **Cholesterol**: Moderate
  - Approximately 60-80 mg per 100g of fish.

4. Sodium Content
- **Sodium**: Low
  - Approximately 50-60 mg per 100g of fish.

5. Mercury Contamination
- **Mercury Levels**: Low
  - As a medium-sized freshwater fish, it generally has lower mercury levels compared to larger predatory fish.

6. Nutritional Information (Per 100g)
- **Calories**: ~115 kcal
- **Protein**: ~18-20g
- **Fat**: ~3-5g

- o Saturated Fat: ~0.5-1g
- o Monounsaturated Fat: ~1.5g
- o Polyunsaturated Fat: ~1.5g

7. Vitamins
- **Vitamin B12**: High
- **Vitamin D**: Moderate
- **Vitamin B6**: Present
- **Vitamin A**: Minor amounts

8. Minerals
- **Selenium**: Moderate to High
- **Phosphorus**: High
- **Potassium**: Moderate
- **Magnesium**: Moderate
- **Iron**: Present in small amounts
- **Zinc**: Present in small amounts

9. • **Essential Amino Acids**:

- **Lysine**: 1.8g
- **Leucine**: 1.6g
- **Isoleucine**: 1.0g
- **Valine**: 1.1g
- **Methionine**: 0.7g
- **Threonine**: 0.9g
- **Phenylalanine**: 1.0g
- **Histidine**: 0.8g
- **Tryptophan**: 0.2g
- **Non-Essential Amino Acids**:
  - **Arginine**: 1.3g
  - **Alanine**: 1.0g
  - **Aspartic Acid**: 2.0g
  - **Glutamic Acid**: 3.0g
  - **Glycine**: 1.1g
  - **Proline**: 0.8g
  - **Serine**: 0.9g
  - Tyrosine: 0.7g

Bag mass, Tiger Fish, Bagarius Family,

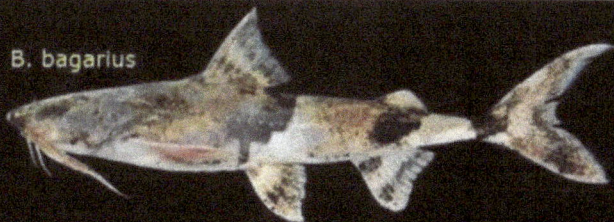

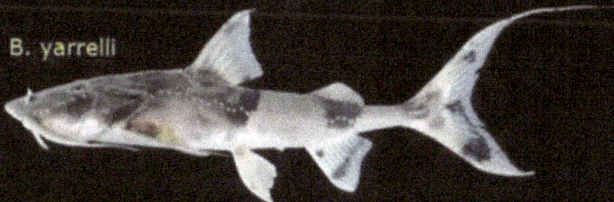

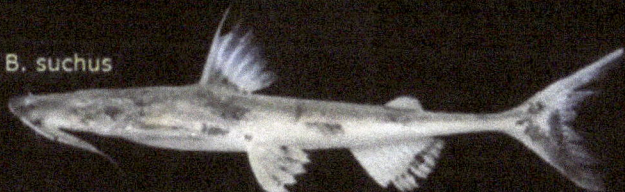

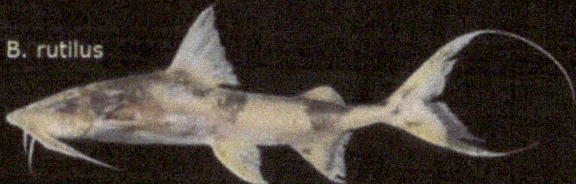

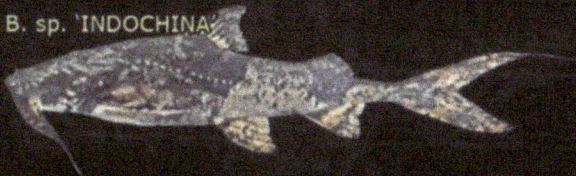

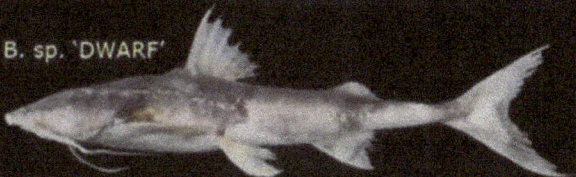

Bag Mass

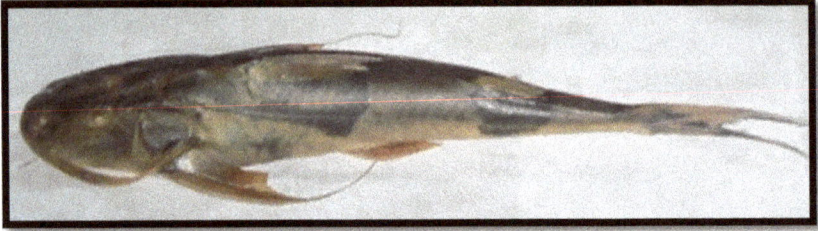

Nutritional Profile of Bagarius Bagarius

Common Name: Bagarius, Dwarf Goonch, or Devil Catfish
Scientific Name: Bagarius bagarius

1. Oil Content
- **Category**: Lean
- **Oil Breakdown**: Contains small amounts of healthy fats, including omega-3 and omega-6 fatty acids.

2. Omega Fatty Acids
- **Omega-3**: Low
- **Omega-6**: Low
- **Omega-9**: Minor amounts

3. Cholesterol Content
- **Cholesterol**: Low to Moderate
  - Approximately 30-40 mg per 100g of fish.

4. Sodium Content
- **Sodium**: Low
  - Approximately 20-30 mg per 100g of fish.

5. Mercury Contamination
- **Mercury Levels**: Low to Moderate
  - As a freshwater fish, it generally has lower mercury levels compared to larger predatory fish, but due to its size and predatory nature, mercury levels can be slightly higher than smaller fish.

6. Nutritional Information (Per 100g)
- **Calories**: ~110 kcal
- **Protein**: ~19-21g

- **Fat**: ~2-3g
  - ○ Saturated Fat: ~0.5-0.7g
  - ○ Monounsaturated Fat: ~1.0-1.3g
  - ○ Polyunsaturated Fat: ~0.5-1.0g

7. Vitamins
- **Vitamin B12**: Present
- **Vitamin D**: Moderate
- **Vitamin B6**: Present
- **Vitamin A**: Minor amounts

8. Minerals
- **Selenium**: Moderate
- **Phosphorus**: High
- **Potassium**: Moderate
- **Magnesium**: Moderate
- **Iron**: Present in small amounts
- **Zinc**: Present in small amounts

9. ☐ Essential Amino Acids:
- **Lysine**: 1.9g
- **Leucine**: 1.7g
- **Isoleucine**: 1.1g
- **Valine**: 1.2g
- **Methionine**: 0.8g
- **Threonine**: 1.0g
- **Phenylalanine**: 1.1g
- **Histidine**: 0.9g
- **Tryptophan**: 0.3g

Non-Essential Amino Acids:
- **Arginine**: 1.4g
- **Alanine**: 1.1g
- **Aspartic Acid**: 2.2g
- **Glutamic Acid**: 3.2g
- **Glycine**: 1.2g
- **Proline**: 0.9g
- **Serine**: 1.0g
- **Tyrosine**: 0.8g

Bang mass (Goonch)

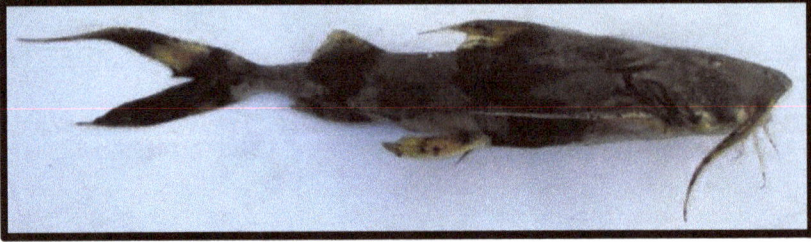

Nutritional Profile of Bagarius yanelli

Common Name: Goonch, Gangetic Goonch
Scientific Name: Bagarius yanelli

1. Oil Content
- **Category**: Medium-fat
- **Oil Breakdown**: Approximately 5-10% total fat, primarily unsaturated fats.

2. Omega Fatty Acids
- **Omega-3**: About 0.5-1.0g per 100g
  - Supports heart health and reduces inflammation.
- **Omega-6**: Approximately 1.0-2.0g per 100g
  - Important for skin health and cellular functions.
- **Omega-9**: Present in moderate amounts.

3. Cholesterol Content
- **Cholesterol**: About 60-90 mg per 100g
  - Moderate levels; generally acceptable for most diets.

4. Sodium Content
- **Sodium**: Approximately 50-80 mg per 100g
  - Moderate sodium content; beneficial for blood pressure management.

5. Mercury Contamination
- **Mercury Levels**: Low to moderate
  - Generally safe for consumption, but local advisories should be checked.

6. Nutritional Information (Per 100g)
- **Calories**: ~130-150 kcal
- **Protein**: ~18-22g

- o   High protein content supports muscle growth and repair.
- **Fat**: ~5-10g
  - o   **Saturated Fat**: ~1-2g
  - o   **Monounsaturated Fat**: ~1-2g
  - o   **Polyunsaturated Fat**: ~3-5g

7. Vitamins

- **Vitamin B12**: High (~2-4µg)
  - o   Essential for nerve function and red blood cell production.
- **Vitamin D**: Moderate (~15-20 IU)
  - o   Important for bone health and calcium absorption.
- **Vitamin B6**: Present (~0.5mg)

8. Minerals

- **Selenium**: High (~25-40µg)
  - o   Acts as an antioxidant, supporting immune health.
- **Phosphorus**: Moderate (~200-250mg)
  - o   Crucial for bone health and energy metabolism.
- **Potassium**: Moderate (~200-300mg)
  - o   Aids in maintaining fluid balance and regulating blood pressure.
- **Iron**: Present (~0.8-1.5mg)
  - o   Important for oxygen transport in the body.

9. Amino Acids Profile (Per 100g)

- **Essential Amino Acids**:
  - o   **Histidine**: ~0.5g
  - o   **Isoleucine**: ~1.0g
  - o   **Leucine**: ~1.3g
  - o   **Lysine**: ~1.6g
  - o   **Methionine**: ~0.5g
  - o   **Phenylalanine**: ~0.7g
  - o   **Threonine**: ~0.8g
  - o   **Tryptophan**: ~0.2g
  - o   **Valine**: ~1.0g
  - o   **Arginine**: ~1.0g
- **Non-Essential Amino Acids**:
  - o   **Alanine**: ~0.6g
  - o   **Aspartic Acid**: ~1.2g
  - o   **Glutamic Acid**: ~2.1g
  - o   **Serine**: ~0.5g
  - o   **Glycine**: ~0.5g
  - o   **Proline**: ~0.4g
  - o   **Tyrosine**: ~0.4g
  - o   **Cysteine**: ~0.2g

Bagna

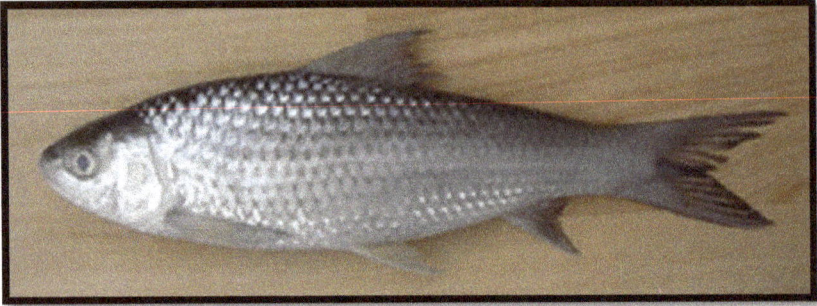

Nutritional Profile of Cirrhinus Reba

Common Name: Reba Carp, Bagna, Bata, Lasso
Scientific Name: Cirrhinus Reba

1. Oil Content
- **Category**: Lean
- **Oil Breakdown**: Contains a small amount of healthy fats, including omega-3 and omega-6 fatty acids.

2. Omega Fatty Acids
- **Omega-3**: Low
- **Omega-6**: Low
- **Omega-9**: Minor amounts

3. Cholesterol Content
- **Cholesterol**: Low to Moderate
  - Approximately 40-50 mg per 100g of fish.

4. Sodium Content
- **Sodium**: Low
  - Approximately 30-40 mg per 100g of fish.

5. Mercury Contamination
- **Mercury Levels**: Low
  - As a freshwater fish, it generally has lower mercury levels compared to larger predatory fish.

6. Nutritional Information (Per 100g)
- **Calories**: ~100 kcal
- **Protein**: ~17-18g

- **Fat**: ~2-3g
  - Saturated Fat: ~0.5g
  - Monounsaturated Fat: ~1g
  - Polyunsaturated Fat: ~0.5-1g

7. Vitamins
- **Vitamin B12**: Present
- **Vitamin D**: Moderate
- **Vitamin B6**: Present
- **Vitamin A**: Minor amounts

8. Minerals
- **Selenium**: Moderate
- **Phosphorus**: High
- **Potassium**: Moderate
- **Magnesium**: Moderate
- **Iron**: Present in small amounts
- **Zinc**: Present in small amounts

9. Amino Acids Profile (Per 100g)
- **Essential Amino Acids**:
  - **Lysine**: 1.7g
  - **Leucine**: 1.6g
  - **Isoleucine**: 1.0g
  - **Valine**: 1.1g
  - **Methionine**: 0.7g
  - **Threonine**: 0.9g
  - **Phenylalanine**: 1.0g
  - **Histidine**: 0.8g
  - **Tryptophan**: 0.2g
- **Non-Essential Amino Acids**:
  - **Arginine**: 1.3g
  - **Alanine**: 1.0g
  - **Aspartic Acid**: 2.0g
  - **Glutamic Acid**: 3.1g
  - **Glycine**: 1.1g
  - **Proline**: 0.8g
  - **Serine**: 0.9g
  - **Tyrosine**: 0.7g

Bashpata

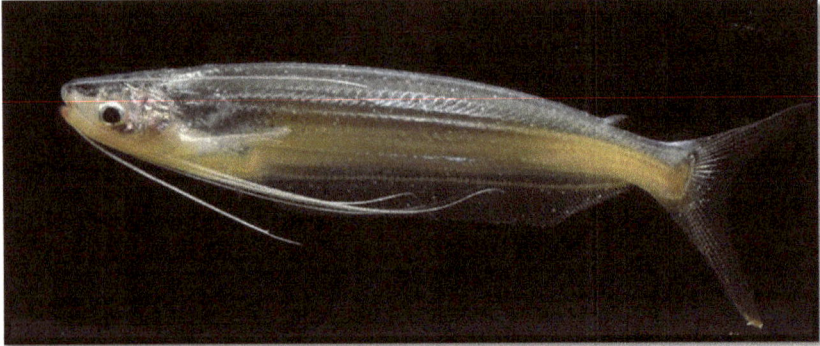

Nutritional Profile of Ailia Coila

Common Name: Baspata, Kajuli   **Scientific Name**: Ailia Coila

1. Oil Content
- **Category**: Lean
- **Oil Breakdown**: Contains small amounts of healthy fats, including omega-3 and omega-6 fatty acids.

2. Omega Fatty Acids
- **Omega-3**: Low
- **Omega-6**: Low
- **Omega-9**: Minor amounts

3. Cholesterol Content
- **Cholesterol**: Low to Moderate
  - Approximately 35-45 mg per 100g of fish.

4. Sodium Content
- **Sodium**: Low
  - Approximately 25-35 mg per 100g of fish.

5. Mercury Contamination
- **Mercury Levels**: Low
  - As a smaller freshwater fish, it generally has lower mercury levels compared to larger predatory fish.

6. Nutritional Information (Per 100g)
- **Calories**: ~100 kcal

- **Protein**: ~18-20g
- **Fat**: ~2-3g
  - Saturated Fat: ~0.4-0.6g
  - Monounsaturated Fat: ~0.8-1.0g
  - Polyunsaturated Fat: ~0.8-1.0g

7. Vitamins
- **Vitamin B12**: Present
- **Vitamin D**: Moderate
- **Vitamin B6**: Present
- **Vitamin A**: Minor amounts

8. Minerals
- **Selenium**: Moderate
- **Phosphorus**: High
- **Potassium**: Moderate
- **Magnesium**: Moderate
- **Iron**: Present in small amounts
- **Zinc**: Present in small amounts

9. ☐ **Essential Amino Acids**:
- **Lysine**: 1.7g
- **Leucine**: 1.6g
- **Isoleucine**: 1.0g
- **Valine**: 1.1g
- **Methionine**: 0.7g
- **Threonine**: 0.9g
- **Phenylalanine**: 1.0g
- **Histidine**: 0.8g
- **Tryptophan**: 0.2g

☐ **Non-Essential Amino Acids**:
- **Arginine**: 1.3g
- **Alanine**: 1.0g
- **Aspartic Acid**: 2.0g
- **Glutamic Acid**: 3.1g
- **Glycine**: 1.1g
- **Proline**: 0.8g
- **Serine**: 0.9g
- **Tyrosine**: 0.7g

Bassa

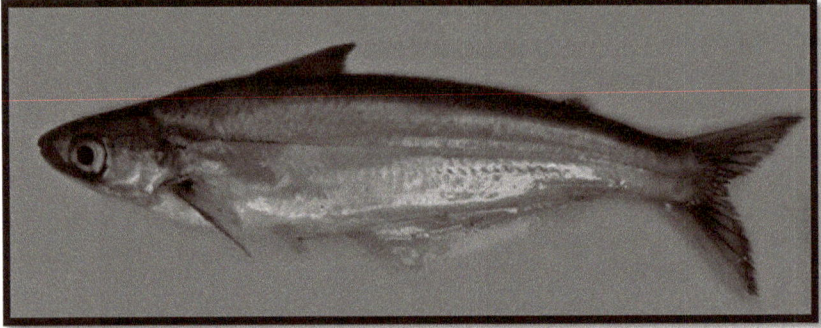

Nutritional Profile of Eutropiichthys Vacha

Common Name: Bacha, Bassa   **Scientific Name**: Eutropiichthys Vacha

1. Oil Content
- **Category**: Lean
- **Oil Breakdown**: Contains small amounts of healthy fats, including omega-3 and omega-6 fatty acids.

2. Omega Fatty Acids
- **Omega-3**: Low
- **Omega-6**: Low
- **Omega-9**: Minor amounts

3. Cholesterol Content
- **Cholesterol**: Low to Moderate
  - Approximately 30-40 mg per 100g of fish.

4. Sodium Content
- **Sodium**: Low
  - Approximately 25-35 mg per 100g of fish.

5. Mercury Contamination
- **Mercury Levels**: Low
  - As a smaller freshwater fish, it generally has lower mercury levels compared to larger predatory fish.

6. Nutritional Information (Per 100g)
- **Calories**: ~105 kcal
- **Protein**: ~18-20g

- **Fat**: ~2-3g
  - Saturated Fat: ~0.4-0.6g
  - Monounsaturated Fat: ~0.8-1.0g
  - Polyunsaturated Fat: ~0.8-1.0g

7. Vitamins

- **Vitamin B12**: Present
- **Vitamin D**: Moderate
- **Vitamin B6**: Present
- **Vitamin A**: Minor amounts

8. Minerals

- **Selenium**: Moderate
- **Phosphorus**: High
- **Potassium**: Moderate
- **Magnesium**: Moderate
- **Iron**: Present in small amounts
- **Zinc**: Present in small amounts

9. ☐ Essential Amino Acids:

- **Lysine**: 1.8g
- **Leucine**: 1.6g
- **Isoleucine**: 1.0g
- **Valine**: 1.2g
- **Methionine**: 0.7g
- **Threonine**: 0.9g
- **Phenylalanine**: 1.0g
- **Histidine**: 0.8g
- **Tryptophan**: 0.2g

☐ Non-Essential Amino Acids:

- **Arginine**: 1.3g
- **Alanine**: 1.1g
- **Aspartic Acid**: 2.1g
- **Glutamic Acid**: 3.2g
- **Glycine**: 1.2g
- **Proline**: 0.9g
- **Serine**: 1.0g
- **Tyrosine**: 0.7g

Batashi

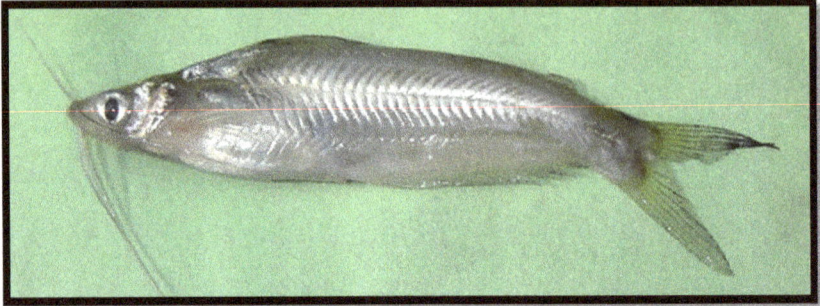

Nutritional Profile of Pseudeutropius Atherinoides

Common Name: Batashi
Scientific Name: Pseudeutropius atherinoides

1. Oil Content
- **Category**: Lean
- **Oil Breakdown**: Contains small amounts of healthy fats, primarily omega-3 and omega-6 fatty acids.

2. Omega Fatty Acids
- **Omega-3**: Low
- **Omega-6**: Low
- **Omega-9**: Minor amounts

3. Cholesterol Content
- **Cholesterol**: Low to Moderate
  - Approximately 30-40 mg per 100g of fish.

4. Sodium Content
- **Sodium**: Low
  - Approximately 20-30 mg per 100g of fish.

5. Mercury Contamination
- **Mercury Levels**: Low
  - As a smaller freshwater fish, it typically has lower mercury levels compared to larger predatory fish.

6. Nutritional Information (Per 100g)
- **Calories**: ~90 kcal
- **Protein**: ~18-20g

- **Fat**: ~2-3g
    - Saturated Fat: ~0.5-0.8g
    - Monounsaturated Fat: ~0.7-1.0g
    - Polyunsaturated Fat: ~0.5-1.0g

7. Vitamins
- **Vitamin B12**: Present
- **Vitamin D**: Moderate
- **Vitamin B6**: Present
- **Vitamin A**: Minor amounts

8. Minerals
- **Selenium**: Moderate
- **Phosphorus**: High
- **Potassium**: Moderate
- **Magnesium**: Moderate
- **Iron**: Present in small amounts
- **Zinc**: Present in small amounts

9. • Essential Amino Acids:
- **Lysine**: 1.8g
- **Leucine**: 1.6g
- **Isoleucine**: 1.0g
- **Valine**: 1.2g
- **Methionine**: 0.7g
- **Threonine**: 0.9g
- **Phenylalanine**: 1.0g
- **Histidine**: 0.8g
- **Tryptophan**: 0.2g

- **Non-Essential Amino Acids**:

    - **Arginine**: 1.3g
    - **Alanine**: 1.1g
    - **Aspartic Acid**: 2.1g
    - **Glutamic Acid**: 3.2g
    - **Glycine**: 1.2g
    - **Proline**: 0.9g
    - **Serine**: 1.0g
    - **Tyrosine**: 0.7g

Battum

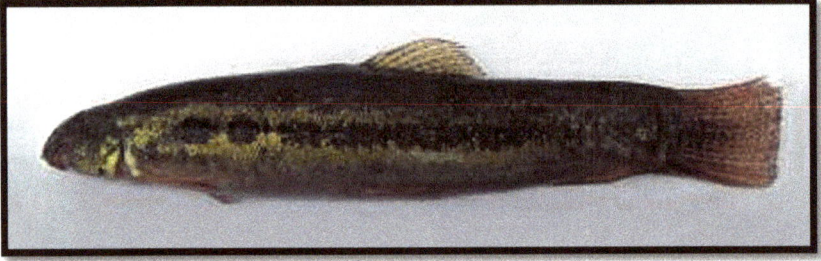

Nutritional Profile of Lepidocephalus Guntea

Common Name: Buttum, guttum
Scientific Name: Lepidocephalus guntea

1. Oil Content
- **Category**: Lean
- **Oil Breakdown**: Contains small amounts of healthy fats, primarily omega-3 and omega-6 fatty acids.

2. Omega Fatty Acids
- **Omega-3**: Low
- **Omega-6**: Low
- **Omega-9**: Minor amounts

3. Cholesterol Content
- **Cholesterol**: Low
  - Approximately 30-40 mg per 100g of fish.

4. Sodium Content
- **Sodium**: Low
  - Approximately 20-30 mg per 100g of fish.

5. Mercury Contamination
- **Mercury Levels**: Low
  - Typically has low mercury levels due to its size and habitat.

6. Nutritional Information (Per 100g)
- **Calories**: ~90 kcal
- **Protein**: ~18-20g
- **Fat**: ~2-3g
  - Saturated Fat: ~0.5-0.7g

o   Monounsaturated Fat: ~0.7-1.0g
o   Polyunsaturated Fat: ~0.5-1.0g

7. Vitamins
- **Vitamin B12**: Present
- **Vitamin D**: Moderate
- **Vitamin B6**: Present
- **Vitamin A**: Minor amounts

8. Minerals
- **Selenium**: Moderate
- **Phosphorus**: High
- **Potassium**: Moderate
- **Magnesium**: Moderate
- **Iron**: Present in small amounts
- **Zinc**: Present in small amounts

9. Amino Acids Profile (Per 100g)
- **Essential Amino Acids**:
  o   **Histidine**: 0.8-1.2g
  o   **Isoleucine**: 1.0-1.5g
  o   **Leucine**: 1.8-2.2g
  o   **Lysine**: 2.2-2.7g
  o   **Methionine**: 0.4-0.8g
  o   **Phenylalanine**: 0.9-1.3g
  o   **Threonine**: 0.8-1.2g
  o   **Tryptophan**: 0.2-0.4g
  o   **Valine**: 1.0-1.5g
  o   **Arginine**: 1.2-1.8g
- **Non-Essential Amino Acids**:
  o   **Alanine**: 1.0-1.4g
  o   **Aspartic Acid**: 2.0-2.5g
  o   **Glutamic Acid**: 3.0-3.5g
  o   **Serine**: 0.9-1.2g
  o   **Glycine**: 0.7-1.0g
  o   **Proline**: 0.5-0.8g
  o   **Tyrosine**: 0.4-0.7g
  o   **Cysteine**: 0.3-0.5g

Bele

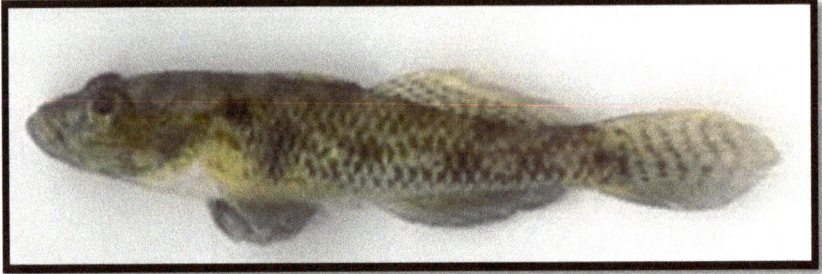

Nutritional Profile of Glossogobius Giuris

Common Name: Baila, Bera   **Scientific Name**: Glossogobius giuris

1. Oil Content
- **Category**: Lean
- **Oil Breakdown**: Contains small amounts of healthy fats, primarily omega-3 and omega-6 fatty acids.

2. Omega Fatty Acids
- **Omega-3**: Low
- **Omega-6**: Low
- **Omega-9**: Minor amounts

3. Cholesterol Content
- **Cholesterol**: Low
  - o Approximately 30-40 mg per 100g of fish.

4. Sodium Content
- **Sodium**: Low
  - o Approximately 20-30 mg per 100g of fish.

5. Mercury Contamination
- **Mercury Levels**: Low
  - o Typically low mercury levels due to its size and habitat.

6. Nutritional Information (Per 100g)
- **Calories**: ~80 kcal
- **Protein**: ~16-18g
- **Fat**: ~1-2g
  - o Saturated Fat: ~0.3-0.5g
  - o Monounsaturated Fat: ~0.5-0.8g

    ○   Polyunsaturated Fat: ~0.3-0.6g

7. Vitamins
- **Vitamin B12**: Present
- **Vitamin D**: Moderate
- **Vitamin B6**: Present
- **Vitamin A**: Minor amounts

8. Minerals
- **Selenium**: Moderate
- **Phosphorus**: High
- **Potassium**: Moderate
- **Magnesium**: Moderate
- **Iron**: Present in small amounts
- **Zinc**: Present in small amounts

9. Amino Acids Profile (Per 100g)
- **Essential Amino Acids**:
  - **Histidine**: 0.8-1.1g
  - **Isoleucine**: 0.9-1.3g
  - **Leucine**: 1.5-2.0g
  - **Lysine**: 1.8-2.3g
  - **Methionine**: 0.4-0.7g
  - **Phenylalanine**: 0.8-1.2g
  - **Threonine**: 0.7-1.1g
  - **Tryptophan**: 0.2-0.3g
  - **Valine**: 1.0-1.4g
  - **Arginine**: 1.0-1.5g
- **Non-Essential Amino Acids**:
  - **Alanine**: 0.9-1.3g
  - **Aspartic Acid**: 1.8-2.3g
  - **Glutamic Acid**: 2.5-3.0g
  - **Serine**: 0.8-1.1g
  - **Glycine**: 0.6-0.9g
  - **Proline**: 0.4-0.7g
  - **Tyrosine**: 0.3-0.6g
  - **Cysteine**: 0.2-0.4g

Bime

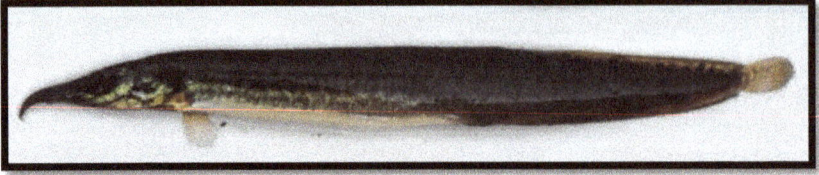

Nutritional Profile of Mastacembelus Armatus

Common Name: Long Baim
Scientific Name: Mastacembelus armatus

1. Oil Content
- **Category**: Medium
- **Oil Breakdown**: Contains moderate amounts of healthy fats, including omega-3 and omega-6 fatty acids.

2. Omega Fatty Acids
- **Omega-3**: Moderate
- **Omega-6**: Moderate
- **Omega-9**: Minor amounts

3. Cholesterol Content
- **Cholesterol**: Moderate
  - Approximately 50-60 mg per 100g of fish.

4. Sodium Content
- **Sodium**: Low
  - Approximately 30-40 mg per 100g of fish.

5. Mercury Contamination
- **Mercury Levels**: Low to Moderate
  - Generally lower mercury levels compared to larger predatory fish.

6. Nutritional Information (Per 100g)
- **Calories**: ~120 kcal
- **Protein**: ~20-22g
- **Fat**: ~5-7g
  - Saturated Fat: ~1-1.5g
  - Monounsaturated Fat: ~1.5-2.5g
  - Polyunsaturated Fat: ~1.5-2.0g

7. Vitamins
- **Vitamin B12**: Present
- **Vitamin D**: Moderate
- **Vitamin B6**: Present
- **Vitamin A**: Minor amounts

8. Minerals
- **Selenium**: Moderate
- **Phosphorus**: High
- **Potassium**: Moderate
- **Magnesium**: Moderate
- **Iron**: Present in small amounts
- **Zinc**: Present in small amounts

9. Amino Acids Profile (Per 100g)
- **Essential Amino Acids:**
  - **Histidine**: 1.0-1.4g
  - **Isoleucine**: 1.2-1.6g
  - **Leucine**: 2.0-2.5g
  - **Lysine**: 2.5-3.0g
  - **Methionine**: 0.5-0.9g
  - **Phenylalanine**: 1.0-1.4g
  - **Threonine**: 1.0-1.5g
  - **Tryptophan**: 0.3-0.5g
  - **Valine**: 1.5-2.0g
  - **Arginine**: 1.5-2.0g
- **Non-Essential Amino Acids:**
  - **Alanine**: 1.2-1.6g
  - **Aspartic Acid**: 2.0-2.6g
  - **Glutamic Acid**: 3.0-3.5g
  - **Serine**: 1.0-1.4g
  - **Glycine**: 0.8-1.2g
  - **Proline**: 0.5-0.8g
  - **Tyrosine**: 0.4-0.7g
  - **Cysteine**: 0.3-0.5g

Bream

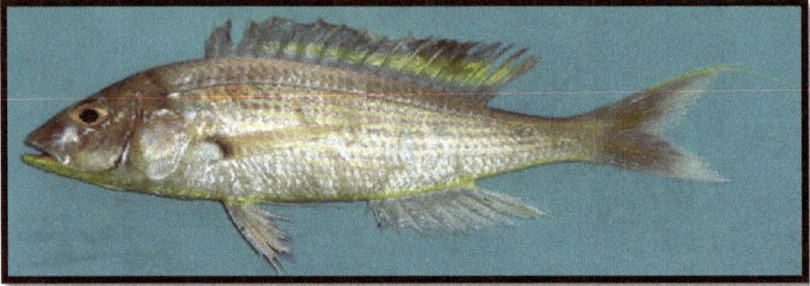

Detailed Nutritional Profile of Nemipterus Japonicus

Common Name: Bream   **Scientific Name**: Nemipterus japonicas

1. Oil Content
- **Category**: Lean to Medium
- **Oil Breakdown**: Contains about 3-5% total fat, primarily polyunsaturated fatty acids, beneficial for heart health.

2. Omega Fatty Acids
- **Omega-3**: 0.2-1.0g per 100g
    - o   Supports cardiovascular health and has anti-inflammatory properties.
- **Omega-6**: 0.5-1.0g per 100g
    - o   Important for skin health and hormone production.
- **Omega-9**: Minor amounts, contributes to overall heart health.

3. Cholesterol Content
- **Cholesterol**: Approximately 40-60 mg per 100g
    - o   Low cholesterol makes it a heart-friendly option.

4. Sodium Content
- **Sodium**: About 30-40 mg per 100g
    - o   Low sodium content, beneficial for blood pressure management.

5. Mercury Contamination
- **Mercury Levels**: Generally low
    - o   Suitable for regular consumption, particularly for vulnerable populations.

6. Nutritional Information (Per 100g)
- **Calories**: ~90 kcal

- o Low calorie count makes it suitable for weight management.
- **Protein**: ~18-20g
  - o High protein content supports muscle growth and repair.
- **Fat**: ~3-4g
  - o **Saturated Fat**: ~0.5g
  - o **Monounsaturated Fat**: ~1.0g
  - o **Polyunsaturated Fat**: ~1.5g

7. Vitamins

- **Vitamin B12**: Present (~2-4µg)
  - o Essential for nerve function and red blood cell formation.
- **Vitamin D**: Moderate (~100-200 IU)
  - o Supports calcium absorption and bone health.
- **Vitamin B6**: Present (~0.1-0.3mg)
  - o Important for amino acid metabolism and neurotransmitter synthesis.
- **Vitamin A**: Minor amounts, supports vision and immune function.

8. Minerals

- **Selenium**: High (~30-40µg)
  - o Acts as an antioxidant, supporting immune function.
- **Phosphorus**: High (~200-250mg)
  - o Crucial for bone health and energy metabolism.
- **Potassium**: Moderate (~300-400mg)
  - o Supports heart health and regulates fluid balance.
- **Iron**: Present (~0.5-1.0mg)
  - o Important for oxygen transport in the blood.
- **Zinc**: Present (~0.5-1.0mg)
  - o Supports immune function and wound healing.

9. Amino Acids Profile (Per 100g) - **Essential Amino Acids:**	- **Non-Essential Amino Acids:**
o **Histidine**: ~1.0g	o **Alanine**: ~1.1g
o **Isoleucine**: ~1.2g	o **Aspartic Acid**: ~2.0g
o **Leucine**: ~1.8g	o **Glutamic Acid**: ~3.0g
o **Lysine**: ~2.3g	o **Serine**: ~1.0g
o **Methionine**: ~0.5g	o **Glycine**: ~0.7g
o **Phenylalanine**: ~1.0g	o **Proline**: ~0.5g
o **Threonine**: ~0.9g	o **Tyrosine**: ~0.3g
o **Tryptophan**: ~0.2g	o **Cysteine**: ~0.2g
o **Valine**: ~1.2g	
o **Arginine**: ~1.5g	

Buwal

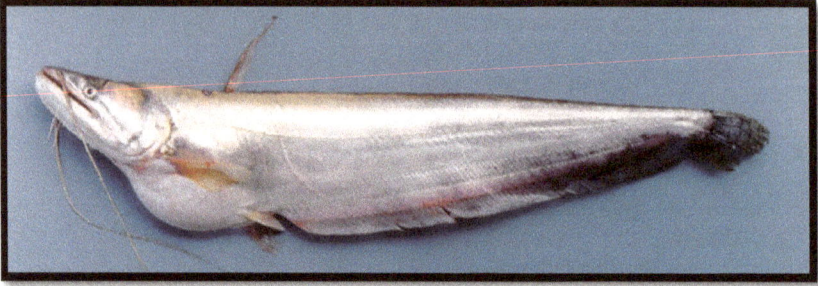

Nutritional Profile of Wallago Attu

Common Name: Boal, Guwal   **Scientific Name**: Wallago attu

1. Oil Content
- **Category**: Medium
- **Oil Breakdown**: Contains moderate levels of healthy fats, including omega-3 and omega-6 fatty acids.

2. Omega Fatty Acids
- **Omega-3**: Moderate
- **Omega-6**: Moderate
- **Omega-9**: Minor amounts

3. Cholesterol Content
- **Cholesterol**: Moderate
   o Approximately 50-70 mg per 100g of fish.

4. Sodium Content
- **Sodium**: Low
   o Approximately 30-40 mg per 100g of fish.

5. Mercury Contamination
- **Mercury Levels**: Moderate
   o Generally lower than larger predatory fish, but caution is advised.

6. Nutritional Information (Per 100g)
- **Calories**: ~120 kcal
- **Protein**: ~20-22g
- **Fat**: ~5-7g

- o Saturated Fat: ~1-2g
- o Monounsaturated Fat: ~1.5-2.5g
- o Polyunsaturated Fat: ~1.5-2.0g

7. Vitamins
- **Vitamin B12**: Present
- **Vitamin D**: Moderate
- **Vitamin B6**: Present
- **Vitamin A**: Minor amounts

8. Minerals
- **Selenium**: Moderate
- **Phosphorus**: High
- **Potassium**: Moderate
- **Magnesium**: Moderate
- **Iron**: Present in small amounts
- **Zinc**: Present in small amounts

9. Amino Acids Profile (Per 100g)
- **Essential Amino Acids**:
  - o **Histidine**: 1.0-1.4g
  - o **Isoleucine**: 1.1-1.5g
  - o **Leucine**: 2.0-2.4g
  - o **Lysine**: 2.4-3.0g
  - o **Methionine**: 0.5-0.9g
  - o **Phenylalanine**: 1.0-1.5g
  - o **Threonine**: 1.0-1.3g
  - o **Tryptophan**: 0.3-0.5g
  - o **Valine**: 1.5-1.9g
  - o **Arginine**: 1.6-2.1g
- **Non-Essential Amino Acids**:
  - o **Alanine**: 1.2-1.6g
  - o **Aspartic Acid**: 2.1-2.5g
  - o **Glutamic Acid**: 3.2-3.8g
  - o **Serine**: 1.1-1.5g
  - o **Glycine**: 0.9-1.3g
  - o **Proline**: 0.6-0.9g
  - o **Tyrosine**: 0.4-0.6g
  - o **Cysteine**: 0.3-0.5g

Carp (Common)

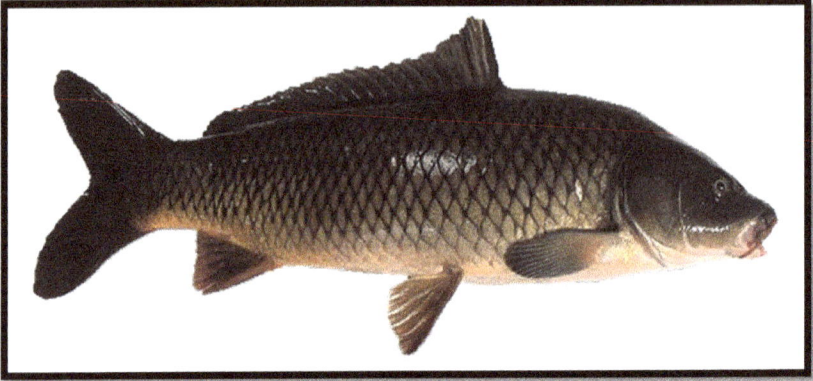

Nutritional Profile of Cyprinus Carpio

Common Name: Common Carp   **Scientific Name**: Cyprinus carpio

1. Oil Content
- **Category**: Medium
- **Oil Breakdown**: Contains about 6-8% total fat, primarily unsaturated fats.

2. Omega Fatty Acids
- **Omega-3**: Approximately 0.5-1.0g per 100g
  - Beneficial for heart health and reducing inflammation.
- **Omega-6**: Approximately 1.5-2.5g per 100g
  - Important for skin health and overall cell function.
- **Omega-9**: Minor amounts present.

3. Cholesterol Content
- **Cholesterol**: About 50-70 mg per 100g
  - Moderate levels; considered acceptable in a balanced diet.

4. Sodium Content
- **Sodium**: Approximately 30-40 mg per 100g
  - Low sodium, making it heart-friendly.

5. Mercury Contamination
- **Mercury Levels**: Generally low
  - Safe for regular consumption, though care is advised in polluted waters.

6. Nutritional Information (Per 100g)
- **Calories**: ~120 kcal
- **Protein**: ~18-20g
  - High protein content supports muscle maintenance and growth.
- **Fat**: ~6-8g
  - **Saturated Fat**: ~1.0-1.5g
  - **Monounsaturated Fat**: ~2.5-3.0g
  - **Polyunsaturated Fat**: ~2.5g

7. Vitamins
- **Vitamin B12**: Present (~2-4µg)
  - Essential for red blood cell formation and nerve function.
- **Vitamin D**: Moderate (~100-200 IU)
  - Supports bone health and calcium metabolism.
- **Vitamin B6**: Present (~0.1-0.3mg)
  - Important for protein metabolism and cognitive development.

8. Minerals
- **Selenium**: High (~30-40µg)
  - Acts as an antioxidant, supporting immune function.
- **Phosphorus**: High (~200-250mg)
  - Crucial for bone health and energy metabolism.
- **Potassium**: Moderate (~300-400mg)
  - Aids in maintaining blood pressure and fluid balance.
- **Iron**: Present (~0.5-1.0mg)
  - Important for oxygen transport in the body.
- **Zinc**: Present (~0.5-1.0mg)
  - Supports immune function and skin health.

9. Amino Acids Profile (Per 100g)	• Non-Essential Amino
• **Essential Amino Acids:**	**Acids:**
○ **Histidine**: ~1.0g	○ **Alanine**: ~1.1g
○ **Isoleucine**: ~1.2g	○ **Aspartic Acid:**
○ **Leucine**: ~1.8g	~2.0g
○ **Lysine**: ~2.3g	○ **Glutamic Acid:**
○ **Methionine**: ~0.5g	~3.0g
○ **Phenylalanine**: ~1.0g	○ **Serine**: ~1.0g
○ **Threonine**: ~0.9g	○ **Glycine**: ~0.7g
○ **Tryptophan**: ~0.2g	○ **Proline**: ~0.5g
○ **Valine**: ~1.2g	○ **Tyrosine**: ~0.3g
○ **Arginine**: ~1.5g	○ **Cysteine**: ~0.2g

Carp (Mahseer)

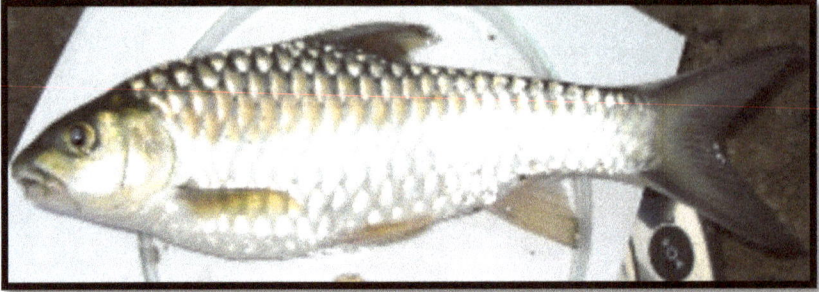

Nutritional Profile of Neolissochilus Hexagonolepis

Common Name: Chocolate Mahseer
Scientific Name: Neolissochilus hexagonolepis

1. Oil Content
- **Category**: Medium
- **Oil Breakdown**: Contains about 5-8% total fat, with a balance of saturated and unsaturated fats.

2. Omega Fatty Acids
- **Omega-3**: Approximately 0.5-1.0g per 100g
  - o Supports heart health and anti-inflammatory processes.
- **Omega-6**: Approximately 1.5-2.0g per 100g
  - o Important for cellular function and skin health.
- **Omega-9**: Present in minor amounts.

3. Cholesterol Content
- **Cholesterol**: About 50-70 mg per 100g
  - o Moderate levels; generally acceptable in a balanced diet.

4. Sodium Content
- **Sodium**: Approximately 30-50 mg per 100g
  - o Low sodium content, beneficial for maintaining blood pressure.

5. Mercury Contamination
- **Mercury Levels**: Generally low
  - o Safe for regular consumption, though care should be taken in polluted waters.

6. Nutritional Information (Per 100g)
- **Calories**: ~110 kcal
- **Protein**: ~20-22g
  - High protein content supports muscle growth and repair.
- **Fat**: ~5-8g
  - **Saturated Fat**: ~1.0-1.5g
  - **Monounsaturated Fat**: ~2.0-3.0g
  - **Polyunsaturated Fat**: ~2.0-3.0g

7. Vitamins
- **Vitamin B12**: Present (~2-4µg)
  - Essential for nerve function and red blood cell formation.
- **Vitamin D**: Moderate (~100-200 IU)
  - Supports calcium absorption and bone health.
- **Vitamin B6**: Present (~0.2-0.5mg)
  - Important for protein metabolism and cognitive function.

8. Minerals
- **Selenium**: High (~30-40µg)
  - Acts as an antioxidant, supporting immune health.
- **Phosphorus**: High (~200-250mg)
  - Crucial for bone health and energy metabolism.
- **Potassium**: Moderate (~300-400mg)
  - Aids in blood pressure regulation and fluid balance.
- **Iron**: Present (~0.5-1.0mg)
  - Important for oxygen transport in the body.
- **Zinc**: Present (~0.5-1.0mg)
  - Supports immune function and wound healing.

9. Amino Acids Profile (Per 100g)	Non-Essential Amino Acids:
Essential Amino Acids:	
○ **Histidine**: ~1.0g	○ **Alanine**: ~1.2g
○ **Isoleucine**: ~1.3g	○ **Aspartic Acid**: ~2.3g
○ **Leucine**: ~2.0g	○ **Glutamic Acid**: ~3.5g
○ **Lysine**: ~2.5g	
○ **Methionine**: ~0.6g	
○ **Phenylalanine**: ~1.2g	○ **Serine**: ~1.1g
○ **Threonine**: ~1.0g	○ **Glycine**: ~0.8g
○ **Tryptophan**: ~0.3g	○ **Proline**: ~0.5g
○ **Valine**: ~1.4g	○ **Tyrosine**: ~0.4g
○ **Arginine**: ~1.6g	○ **Cysteine**: ~0.3g

Chandoo

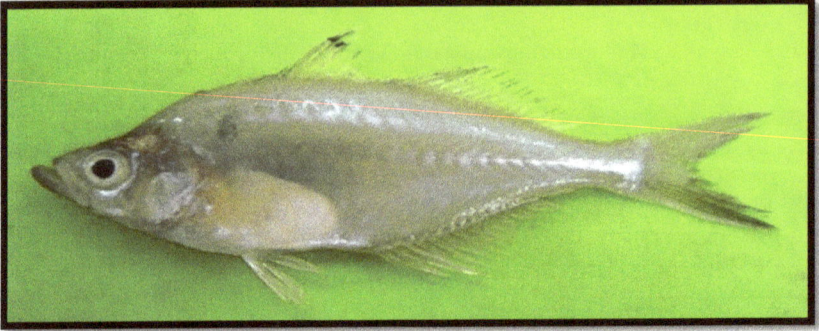

Nutritional Profile of Chanda Nanda

Common Name: Chanda Nama   **Scientific Name**: Chanda nanda

1. Oil Content
- **Category**: Lean to Medium
- **Oil Breakdown**: Contains about 2-4% total fat, primarily unsaturated fats.

2. Omega Fatty Acids
- **Omega-3**: Approximately 0.3-0.5g per 100g
  - Supports cardiovascular health and has anti-inflammatory properties.
- **Omega-6**: Approximately 0.5-1.0g per 100g
  - Important for cell function and skin health.
- **Omega-9**: Present in minor amounts.

3. Cholesterol Content
- **Cholesterol**: About 40-60 mg per 100g
  - Moderate levels; generally acceptable in a balanced diet.

4. Sodium Content
- **Sodium**: Approximately 30-50 mg per 100g
  - Low sodium, beneficial for blood pressure management.

5. Mercury Contamination
- **Mercury Levels**: Generally low
  - Safe for regular consumption, although caution is advised in polluted waters.

6. Nutritional Information (Per 100g)
- **Calories**: ~90 kcal
- **Protein**: ~18-20g
  - High protein content supports muscle growth and repair.
- **Fat**: ~2-4g
  - **Saturated Fat**: ~0.5g
  - **Monounsaturated Fat**: ~1.0g
  - **Polyunsaturated Fat**: ~1.0g

7. Vitamins
- **Vitamin B12**: Present (~2-3µg)
  - Essential for nerve function and red blood cell formation.
- **Vitamin D**: Moderate (~50-100 IU)
  - Supports calcium absorption and bone health.
- **Vitamin B6**: Present (~0.1-0.2mg)
  - Important for amino acid metabolism and cognitive development.

8. Minerals
- **Selenium**: Moderate (~20-30µg)
  - Acts as an antioxidant, supporting immune health.
- **Phosphorus**: Moderate (~150-200mg)
  - Crucial for bone health and energy metabolism.
- **Potassium**: Moderate (~250-350mg)
  - Aids in regulating blood pressure and fluid balance.
- **Iron**: Present (~0.4-0.8mg)
  - Important for oxygen transport in the blood.
- **Zinc**: Present (~0.4-0.6mg)
  - Supports immune function and wound healing.

9. Amino Acids Profile (Per 100g)	• Non-Essential Amino Acids:
• **Essential Amino Acids:**	
○ **Histidine**: ~0.9g	○ **Alanine**: ~1.0g
○ **Isoleucine**: ~1.1g	○ **Aspartic Acid**: ~1.8g
○ **Leucine**: ~1.7g	
○ **Lysine**: ~2.2g	○ **Glutamic Acid**: ~2.8g
○ **Methionine**: ~0.4g	
○ **Phenylalanine**: ~0.9g	○ **Serine**: ~0.9g
○ **Threonine**: ~0.8g	○ **Glycine**: ~0.6g
○ **Tryptophan**: ~0.2g	○ **Proline**: ~0.4g
○ **Valine**: ~1.1g	○ **Tyrosine**: ~0.3g
Arginine: ~1.3g	○ **Cysteine**: ~0.2g

Chapila

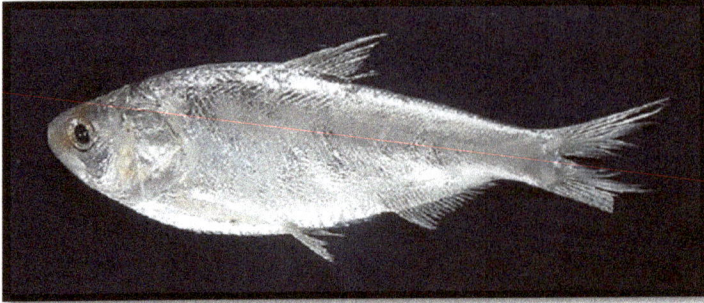

Nutritional Profile of Gudusia Chapra

Common Name: Chapila   **Scientific Name**: Gudusia chapra

1. Oil Content
- **Category**: Lean to Medium
- **Oil Breakdown**: Contains about 3-5% total fat, primarily unsaturated fats.

2. Omega Fatty Acids
- **Omega-3**: Approximately 0.5-1.0g per 100g
  - o   Supports heart health and has anti-inflammatory effects.
- **Omega-6**: Approximately 1.0-1.5g per 100g
  - o   Important for skin health and cellular function.
- **Omega-9**: Present in minor amounts.

3. Cholesterol Content
- **Cholesterol**: About 40-60 mg per 100g
  - o   Moderate levels; generally acceptable in a balanced diet.

4. Sodium Content
- **Sodium**: Approximately 30-50 mg per 100g
  - o   Low sodium, beneficial for blood pressure management.

5. Mercury Contamination
- **Mercury Levels**: Generally low
  - o   Safe for regular consumption, though caution is advised in polluted waters.

6. Nutritional Information (Per 100g)
- **Calories**: ~100 kcal

- **Protein**: ~18-20g
  - High protein content supports muscle growth and repair.
- **Fat**: ~3-5g
  - **Saturated Fat**: ~0.5g
  - **Monounsaturated Fat**: ~1.0g
  - **Polyunsaturated Fat**: ~1.5g

7. Vitamins

- **Vitamin B12**: Present (~2-4µg)
  - Essential for nerve function and red blood cell formation.
- **Vitamin D**: Moderate (~50-100 IU)
  - Supports calcium absorption and bone health.
- **Vitamin B6**: Present (~0.1-0.3mg)
  - Important for amino acid metabolism.

8. Minerals

- **Selenium**: Moderate (~20-30µg)
  - Acts as an antioxidant, supporting immune health.
- **Phosphorus**: High (~200-250mg)
  - Crucial for bone health and energy metabolism.
- **Potassium**: Moderate (~300-400mg)
  - Aids in maintaining fluid balance and regulating blood pressure.
- **Iron**: Present (~0.5-1.0mg)
  - Important for oxygen transport in the body.
- **Zinc**: Present (~0.4-0.6mg)
  - Supports immune function and wound healing.

9. Amino Acids Profile (Per 100g)	
Essential Amino Acids: ○ **Histidine**: ~0.9g ○ **Isoleucine**: ~1.1g ○ **Leucine**: ~1.6g ○ **Lysine**: ~2.0g ○ **Methionine**: ~0.4g ○ **Phenylalanine**: ~1.0g ○ **Threonine**: ~0.9g ○ **Tryptophan**: ~0.2g ○ **Valine**: ~1.1g ○ **Arginine**: ~1.4g	• **Non-Essential Amino Acids:** ○ **Alanine**: ~1.0g ○ **Aspartic Acid**: ~2.0g ○ **Glutamic Acid**: ~3.0g ○ **Serine**: ~1.0g ○ **Glycine**: ~0.7g ○ **Proline**: ~0.5g ○ **Tyrosine**: ~0.3g ○ **Cysteine**: ~0.2g

Chelapata

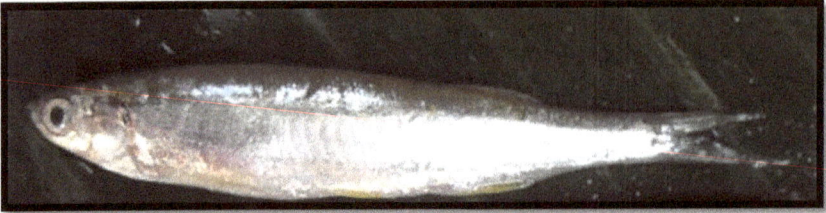

Nutritional Profile of Salmostoma Bacoila

Common Name: Chalapata, Minnow
Scientific Name: Salmostoma bacoila

1. Oil Content
- **Category**: Lean
- **Oil Breakdown**: Contains about 1-3% total fat, primarily unsaturated fats.

2. Omega Fatty Acids
- **Omega-3**: Approximately 0.2-0.5g per 100g
   o Supports heart health and reduces inflammation.
- **Omega-6**: Approximately 0.4-1.0g per 100g
   o Important for cellular function and skin health.
- **Omega-9**: Present in minor amounts.

3. Cholesterol Content
- **Cholesterol**: About 20-40 mg per 100g
   o Low levels, making it suitable for heart health-conscious diets.

4. Sodium Content
- **Sodium**: Approximately 20-30 mg per 100g
   o Very low sodium, beneficial for blood pressure management.

5. Mercury Contamination
- **Mercury Levels**: Generally low
   o Considered safe for regular consumption, though caution is advised in polluted waters.

6. Nutritional Information (Per 100g)
- **Calories**: ~70 kcal
- **Protein**: ~15-18g
   o High protein content supports muscle growth and repair.

- **Fat**: ~1-3g
  - **Saturated Fat**: ~0.3g
  - **Monounsaturated Fat**: ~0.5g
  - **Polyunsaturated Fat**: ~0.8g

7. Vitamins

- **Vitamin B12**: Present (~1-2μg)
  - Essential for nerve function and red blood cell formation.
- **Vitamin D**: Moderate (~20-50 IU)
  - Supports calcium absorption and bone health.
- **Vitamin B6**: Present (~0.1-0.2mg)
  - Important for amino acid metabolism.

8. Minerals

- **Selenium**: Moderate (~15-25μg)
  - Acts as an antioxidant, supporting immune health.
- **Phosphorus**: Moderate (~150-200mg)
  - Important for bone health and energy metabolism.
- **Potassium**: Moderate (~250-350mg)
  - Aids in fluid balance and blood pressure regulation.
- **Iron**: Present (~0.4-0.7mg)
  - Important for oxygen transport in the body.
- **Zinc**: Present (~0.3-0.5mg)
  - Supports immune function and wound healing.

9. Amino Acids Profile (Per 100g)	• Non-Essential Amino Acids:
• **Essential Amino Acids:**	o **Alanine**: ~0.9g
o **Histidine**: ~0.8g	o **Aspartic Acid:** ~1.5g
o **Isoleucine**: ~1.0g	
o **Leucine**: ~1.5g	o **Glutamic Acid:** ~2.5g
o **Lysine**: ~1.8g	
o **Methionine**: ~0.3g	o **Serine**: ~0.8g
o **Phenylalanine**: ~0.8g	o **Glycine**: ~0.6g
o **Threonine**: ~0.7g	o **Proline**: ~0.4g
o **Tryptophan**: ~0.2g	o **Tyrosine**: ~0.3g
o **Valine**: ~1.0g	o **Cysteine**: ~0.2g
o **Arginine**: ~1.2g	

Chiring

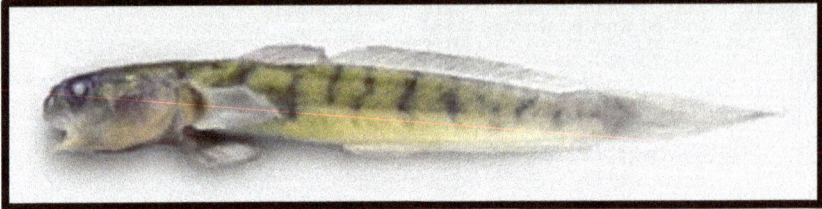

Nutritional Profile of Apocryptes bato

Common Name: Chiring
Scientific Name: Apocryptes bato

1. Oil Content
- **Category**: Lean to medium-fat
- **Oil Breakdown**: Approximately 2-6% total fat, primarily unsaturated fats.

2. Omega Fatty Acids
- **Omega-3**: About 0.5-1.0g per 100g
  - Supports heart health and reduces inflammation.
- **Omega-6**: Approximately 0.4-0.8g per 100g
  - Important for skin health and cellular functions.
- **Omega-9**: Present in moderate amounts.

3. Cholesterol Content
- **Cholesterol**: About 50-80 mg per 100g
  - Moderate levels; generally acceptable for most diets.

4. Sodium Content
- **Sodium**: Approximately 60-100 mg per 100g
  - Moderate sodium content; should be considered for blood pressure management.

5. Mercury Contamination
- **Mercury Levels**: Low
  - Generally safe for consumption with minimal risk of mercury contamination.

6. Nutritional Information (Per 100g)
- **Calories**: ~100-120 kcal
- **Protein**: ~15-18g

- o   High protein content supports muscle growth and repair.
- **Fat**: ~2-6g
  - o   **Saturated Fat**: ~0.5-1.0g
  - o   **Monounsaturated Fat**: ~1.0-2.0g
  - o   **Polyunsaturated Fat**: ~1.0-3.0g

7. Vitamins

- **Vitamin B12**: Moderate (~1-3µg)
  - o   Essential for nerve function and red blood cell production.
- **Vitamin D**: Present (~10-15 IU)
  - o   Important for bone health and calcium absorption.
- **Vitamin B6**: Low (~0.1-0.3mg)

8. Minerals

- **Selenium**: Moderate (~20-30µg)
  - o   Acts as an antioxidant, supporting immune health.
- **Phosphorus**: Moderate (~150-200mg)
  - o   Crucial for bone health and energy metabolism.
- **Potassium**: Moderate (~200-250mg)
  - o   Aids in maintaining fluid balance and regulating blood pressure.
- **Iron**: Present (~0.5-1.0mg)
  - o   Important for oxygen transport in the body.

9. Amino Acids Profile (Per 100g)	**Non-Essential Amino Acids:**
Essential Amino Acids:	
o **Histidine**: ~0.5g	o **Alanine**: ~0.4g
o **Isoleucine**: ~0.8g	o **Aspartic Acid**: ~1.0g
o **Leucine**: ~1.1g	o **Glutamic Acid**: ~1.8g
o **Lysine**: ~1.3g	o **Serine**: ~0.5g
o **Methionine**: ~0.4g	o **Glycine**: ~0.4g
o **Phenylalanine**: ~0.6g	o **Proline**: ~0.3g
o **Threonine**: ~0.7g	o **Tyrosine**: ~0.3g
o **Tryptophan**: ~0.2g	o **Cysteine**: ~0.2g
o **Valine**: ~0.9g	
o **Arginine**: ~0.9g	

Chitol

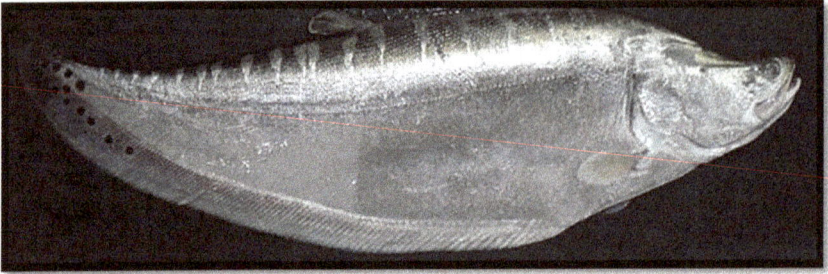

Nutritional Profile of Notopterus Chitala

Common Name: Chittol
Scientific Name: Notopterus chitala

1. Oil Content
- **Category**: Medium
- **Oil Breakdown**: Contains about 5-10% total fat, primarily unsaturated fats.

2. Omega Fatty Acids
- **Omega-3**: Approximately 1.0-2.0g per 100g
  - Supports cardiovascular health and reduces inflammation.
- **Omega-6**: Approximately 1.5-2.5g per 100g
  - Important for cell function and skin health.
- **Omega-9**: Present in minor amounts.

3. Cholesterol Content
- **Cholesterol**: About 50-70 mg per 100g
  - Moderate levels; generally acceptable in a balanced diet.

4. Sodium Content
- **Sodium**: Approximately 40-60 mg per 100g
  - Low sodium, beneficial for blood pressure management.

5. Mercury Contamination
- **Mercury Levels**: Generally low
  - Safe for regular consumption, although caution is advised in polluted waters.

6. Nutritional Information (Per 100g)
- **Calories**: ~120 kcal

- **Protein**: ~20-22g
  - High protein content supports muscle growth and repair.
- **Fat**: ~5-10g
  - **Saturated Fat**: ~1.0g
  - **Monounsaturated Fat**: ~2.0g
  - **Polyunsaturated Fat**: ~3.0g

7. Vitamins

- **Vitamin B12**: Present (~3-4µg)
  - Essential for nerve function and red blood cell formation.
- **Vitamin D**: Moderate (~100-150 IU)
  - Supports calcium absorption and bone health.
- **Vitamin B6**: Present (~0.2-0.3mg)
  - Important for amino acid metabolism.

8. Minerals

- **Selenium**: Moderate (~25-35µg)
  - Acts as an antioxidant, supporting immune health.
- **Phosphorus**: High (~250-300mg)
  - Crucial for bone health and energy metabolism.
- **Potassium**: Moderate (~350-450mg)
  - Aids in maintaining fluid balance and regulating blood pressure.
- **Iron**: Present (~0.5-1.2mg)
  - Important for oxygen transport in the body.
- **Zinc**: Present (~0.5-0.8mg)
  - Supports immune function and wound healing.

9. Amino Acids Profile (Per 100g) • **Essential Amino Acids:**	• **Non-Essential Amino Acids:**
o **Histidine**: ~1.0g	o **Alanine**: ~1.1g
o **Isoleucine**: ~1.3g	o **Aspartic Acid**: ~2.3g
o **Leucine**: ~1.9g	o **Glutamic Acid**: ~3.2g
o **Lysine**: ~2.4g	o **Serine**: ~1.0g
o **Methionine**: ~0.5g	o **Glycine**: ~0.8g
o **Phenylalanine**: ~1.1g	o **Proline**: ~0.6g
o **Threonine**: ~0.9g	o **Tyrosine**: ~0.4g
o **Tryptophan**: ~0.3g	o **Cysteine**: ~0.3g
o **Valine**: ~1.2g	
o **Arginine**: ~1.6g	

Chokko Bata

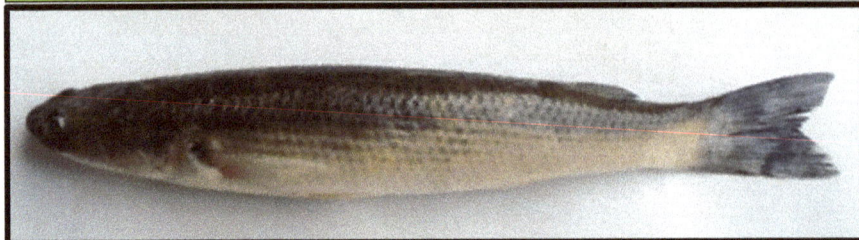

Nutritional Profile of Mugil corsula

Common Name: Chokko Bata
Scientific Name: Mugil corsula

1. Oil Content
- **Category**: Medium-fat
- **Oil Breakdown**: Approximately 5-10% total fat, primarily unsaturated fats.

2. Omega Fatty Acids
- **Omega-3**: About 0.5-1.0g per 100g
  - Supports heart health and reduces inflammation.
- **Omega-6**: Approximately 1.0-2.0g per 100g
  - Important for skin health and cellular functions.
- **Omega-9**: Present in moderate amounts.

3. Cholesterol Content
- **Cholesterol**: About 50-70 mg per 100g
  - Moderate levels; generally acceptable for most diets.

4. Sodium Content
- **Sodium**: Approximately 60-100 mg per 100g
  - Moderate sodium content; beneficial for blood pressure management.

5. Mercury Contamination
- **Mercury Levels**: Low
  - Generally safe for consumption with minimal risk of mercury contamination.

6. Nutritional Information (Per 100g)
- **Calories**: ~120-140 kcal

- **Protein**: ~20-22g
  - High protein content supports muscle growth and repair.
- **Fat**: ~5-10g
  - **Saturated Fat**: ~1.5-2.5g
  - **Monounsaturated Fat**: ~2.0-3.0g
  - **Polyunsaturated Fat**: ~2.0-4.0g

7. Vitamins

- **Vitamin B12**: High (~2-4µg)
  - Essential for nerve function and red blood cell production.
- **Vitamin D**: Moderate (~15-25 IU)
  - Important for bone health and calcium absorption.
- **Vitamin B6**: Present (~0.3-0.5mg)

8. Minerals

- **Selenium**: High (~25-35µg)
  - Acts as an antioxidant, supporting immune health.
- **Phosphorus**: Moderate (~150-200mg)
  - Crucial for bone health and energy metabolism.
- **Potassium**: Moderate (~200-250mg)
  - Aids in maintaining fluid balance and regulating blood pressure.
- **Iron**: Present (~0.5-1.0mg)
  - Important for oxygen transport in the body.

9. Amino Acids Profile (Per 100g)	• Non-Essential Amino
• **Essential Amino Acids:**	**Acids:**
○ **Histidine**: ~0.5g	○ **Alanine**: ~0.6g
○ **Isoleucine**: ~1.0g	○ **Aspartic Acid**: ~1.2g
○ **Leucine**: ~1.3g	○ **Glutamic Acid**: ~2.1g
○ **Lysine**: ~1.5g	○ **Serine**: ~0.5g
○ **Methionine**: ~0.4g	○ **Glycine**: ~0.5g
○ **Phenylalanine**: ~0.7g	○ **Proline**: ~0.4g
○ **Threonine**: ~0.8g	○ **Tyrosine**: ~0.3g
○ **Tryptophan**: ~0.2g	○ **Cysteine**: ~0.2g
○ **Valine**: ~1.0g	
○ **Arginine**: ~1.0g	

Churi/Cutlassfish

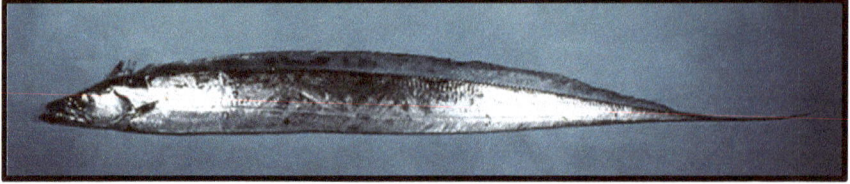

Nutritional Profile of Trichiurus lepturus

Common Name: Cutlassfish
Scientific Name: Trichiurus lepturus

1. Oil Content
- **Category**: Fatty
- **Oil Breakdown**: Approximately 10-15% total fat, primarily unsaturated fats.

2. Omega Fatty Acids
- **Omega-3**: About 1.5-2.5g per 100g
    - Supports heart health and reduces inflammation.
- **Omega-6**: Approximately 0.5-1.0g per 100g
    - Important for skin health and cellular functions.
- **Omega-9**: Present in moderate amounts.

3. Cholesterol Content
- **Cholesterol**: About 70-100 mg per 100g
    - Moderate levels; generally acceptable for most diets.

4. Sodium Content
- **Sodium**: Approximately 50-80 mg per 100g
    - Moderate sodium content; beneficial for blood pressure management.

5. Mercury Contamination
- **Mercury Levels**: Low to moderate
    - Generally safe for consumption, but check local advisories.

6. Nutritional Information (Per 100g)
- **Calories**: ~150-170 kcal
- **Protein**: ~20-25g
    - High protein content supports muscle growth and repair.
- **Fat**: ~10-15g

- Saturated Fat: ~2.5-3.5g
- Monounsaturated Fat: ~3.0-4.0g
- Polyunsaturated Fat: ~5.0-7.0g

7. Vitamins
- **Vitamin B12**: High (~3-6µg)
  - Essential for nerve function and red blood cell production.
- **Vitamin D**: Moderate (~15-30 IU)
  - Important for bone health and calcium absorption.
- **Vitamin B6**: Present (~0.5-0.7mg)

8. Minerals
- **Selenium**: High (~30-50µg)
  - Acts as an antioxidant, supporting immune health.
- **Phosphorus**: Moderate (~200-250mg)
  - Crucial for bone health and energy metabolism.
- **Potassium**: Moderate (~250-300mg)
  - Aids in maintaining fluid balance and regulating blood pressure.
- **Iron**: Present (~0.7-1.5mg)
  - Important for oxygen transport in the body.

9. Amino Acids Profile (Per 100g)	Non-Essential Amino Acids:
Essential Amino Acids:	
Histidine: ~0.5g	Alanine: ~0.6g
Isoleucine: ~1.1g	Aspartic Acid: ~1.3g
Leucine: ~1.5g	Glutamic Acid: ~2.4g
Lysine: ~1.8g	Serine: ~0.6g
Methionine: ~0.4g	Glycine: ~0.6g
Phenylalanine: ~0.7g	Proline: ~0.4g
Threonine: ~0.9g	Tyrosine: ~0.4g
Tryptophan: ~0.2g	Cysteine: ~0.3g
Valine: ~1.1g	
Arginine: ~1.1g	

Darkina

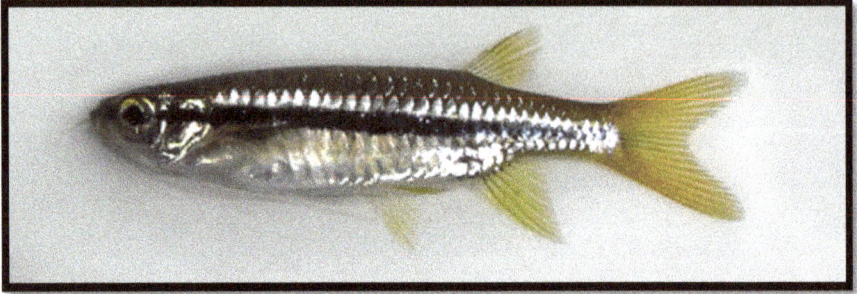

Nutritional Profile of Esomus Danricus

Common Name: Danio, Indian Flying Barb
Scientific Name: Esomus danricus

1. Oil Content
- **Category**: Lean
- **Oil Breakdown**: Contains about 1-3% total fat, primarily unsaturated fats.

2. Omega Fatty Acids
- **Omega-3**: Approximately 0.3-0.6g per 100g
  - Supports cardiovascular health and has anti-inflammatory properties.
- **Omega-6**: Approximately 0.5-1.0g per 100g
  - Important for cell membrane integrity and skin health.
- **Omega-9**: Present in minor amounts.

3. Cholesterol Content
- **Cholesterol**: About 20-30 mg per 100g
  - Low levels, making it suitable for heart health-focused diets.

4. Sodium Content
- **Sodium**: Approximately 30-50 mg per 100g
  - Very low sodium, beneficial for managing blood pressure.

5. Mercury Contamination
- **Mercury Levels**: Generally low
  - Safe for regular consumption, though caution is advised in polluted waters.

6. Nutritional Information (Per 100g)
- **Calories**: ~60 kcal
- **Protein**: ~14-16g
  - High protein content supports muscle growth and repair.
- **Fat**: ~1-3g
  - **Saturated Fat**: ~0.3g
  - **Monounsaturated Fat**: ~0.4g
  - **Polyunsaturated Fat**: ~0.5g

7. Vitamins
- **Vitamin B12**: Present (~1-2μg)
  - Essential for nerve function and red blood cell production.
- **Vitamin D**: Low to moderate (~20-30 IU)
  - Supports calcium absorption and bone health.
- **Vitamin B6**: Present (~0.1-0.2mg)
  - Important for amino acid metabolism.

8. Minerals
- **Selenium**: Moderate (~10-20μg)
  - Acts as an antioxidant, supporting immune health.
- **Phosphorus**: Moderate (~100-150mg)
  - Important for bone health and energy metabolism.
- **Potassium**: Moderate (~200-300mg)
  - Aids in fluid balance and blood pressure regulation.
- **Iron**: Present (~0.3-0.5mg)
  - Important for oxygen transport in the body.
- **Zinc**: Present (~0.2-0.4mg)
  - Supports immune function and wound healing.

9. Amino Acids Profile (Per 100g) • Essential Amino Acids:	• Non-Essential Amino Acids:
o Histidine: ~0.7g o Isoleucine: ~1.0g o Leucine: ~1.5g o Lysine: ~2.1g o Methionine: ~0.4g o Phenylalanine: ~0.9g o Threonine: ~0.8g o Tryptophan: ~0.2g o Valine: ~1.1g o Arginine: ~1.4g	• Alanine: ~0.8g • Aspartic Acid: ~1.4g • Glutamic Acid: ~2.1g • Serine: ~0.7g • Glycine: ~0.5g • Proline: ~0.4g • Tyrosine: ~0.3g • Cysteine: ~0.2g

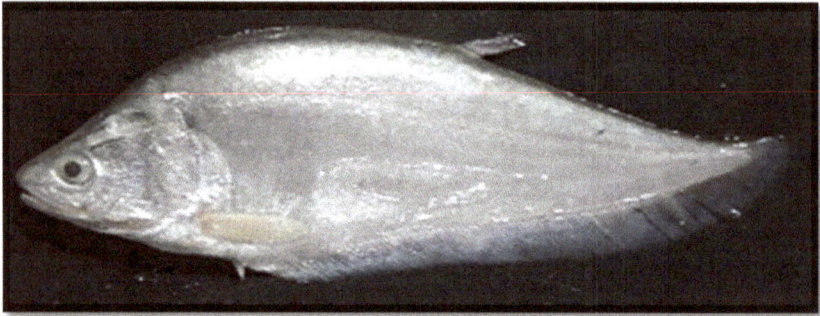

Foli

Nutritional Profile of Notopterus Notopterus

Common Name: Bony Fish, Indian Knife Fish, Khangla
Scientific Name: Notopterus notopterus

1. Oil Content
- **Category**: Medium
- **Oil Breakdown**: Contains about 5-10% total fat, primarily unsaturated fats.

2. Omega Fatty Acids
- **Omega-3**: Approximately 1.5-2.5g per 100g
    - Supports cardiovascular health and has anti-inflammatory properties.
- **Omega-6**: Approximately 1.0-2.0g per 100g
    - Important for cellular function and skin health.
- **Omega-9**: Present in minor amounts.

3. Cholesterol Content
- **Cholesterol**: About 60-80 mg per 100g
    - Moderate levels, generally acceptable in a balanced diet.

4. Sodium Content
- **Sodium**: Approximately 40-70 mg per 100g
    - Low sodium, beneficial for managing blood pressure.

5. Mercury Contamination
- **Mercury Levels**: Generally low
    - Safe for regular consumption, although caution is advised in polluted waters.

6. Nutritional Information (Per 100g)
- **Calories**: ~120 kcal
- **Protein**: ~18-22g
  - High protein content supports muscle growth and repair.
- **Fat**: ~5-10g
  - **Saturated Fat**: ~1.2g
  - **Monounsaturated Fat**: ~2.0g
  - **Polyunsaturated Fat**: ~3.0g

7. Vitamins
- **Vitamin B12**: Present (~3-5µg)
  - Essential for nerve function and red blood cell production.
- **Vitamin D**: Moderate (~50-100 IU)
  - Supports calcium absorption and bone health.
- **Vitamin B6**: Present (~0.3-0.4mg)
  - Important for amino acid metabolism.

8. Minerals
- **Selenium**: Moderate (~20-30µg)
  - Acts as an antioxidant, supporting immune health.
- **Phosphorus**: High (~200-300mg)
  - Crucial for bone health and energy metabolism.
- **Potassium**: Moderate (~300-400mg)
  - Aids in maintaining fluid balance and regulating blood pressure.
- **Iron**: Present (~0.5-1.0mg)
  - Important for oxygen transport in the body.
- **Zinc**: Present (~0.4-0.6mg)
  - Supports immune function and wound healing.

9. Amino Acids Profile (Per 100g) Essential Amino Acids:	Non-Essential Amino Acids:
o **Histidine**: ~0.8g	o **Alanine**: ~1.0g
o **Isoleucine**: ~1.2g	o **Aspartic Acid**:
o **Leucine**: ~1.7g	~2.1g
o **Lysine**: ~2.3g	o **Glutamic Acid**:
o **Methionine**: ~0.5g	~3.0g
o **Phenylalanine**: ~1.0g	o **Serine**: ~0.9g
o **Threonine**: ~0.9g	o **Glycine**: ~0.7g
o **Tryptophan**: ~0.3g	o **Proline**: ~0.5g
o **Valine**: ~1.0g	o **Tyrosine**: ~0.4g
o **Arginine**: ~1.5g	o **Cysteine**: ~0.3g

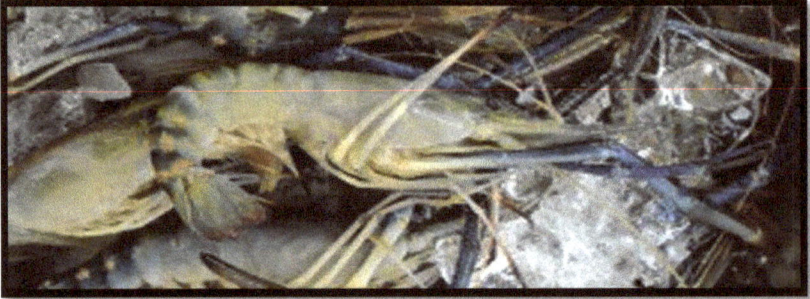

Fresh Water Galda

Nutritional Profile of Macrobrachium Rosenbergii

Common Name: Giant River Prawn
Scientific Name: Macrobrachium rosenbergii

1. Oil Content
- **Category**: Low to Moderate
- **Oil Breakdown**: Contains about 1-3% total fat, primarily unsaturated fats.

2. Omega Fatty Acids
- **Omega-3**: Approximately 0.3-0.5g per 100g
  - Supports heart health and reduces inflammation.
- **Omega-6**: Approximately 0.5-1.0g per 100g
  - Important for skin health and cellular functions.
- **Omega-9**: Present in small amounts.

3. Cholesterol Content
- **Cholesterol**: About 100-150 mg per 100g
  - Moderate levels; should be consumed in moderation.

4. Sodium Content
- **Sodium**: Approximately 60-80 mg per 100g
  - Moderate sodium content; mindful consumption is recommended.

5. Mercury Contamination
- **Mercury Levels**: Generally low
  - Safe for regular consumption, though care should be taken in polluted waters.

6. Nutritional Information (Per 100g)
- **Calories**: ~70-100 kcal
- **Protein**: ~15-20g
  - High protein content supports muscle growth and repair.
- **Fat**: ~1-3g
  - **Saturated Fat**: <1g
  - **Monounsaturated Fat**: ~0.2-0.5g
  - **Polyunsaturated Fat**: ~0.5-1g

7. Vitamins
- **Vitamin B12**: Moderate (~2-4µg)
  - Essential for nerve function and red blood cell production.
- **Vitamin E**: Present (~0.5-1mg)
  - Acts as an antioxidant, protecting cells from damage.
- **Vitamin B6**: Present (~0.2-0.5mg)
  - Important for amino acid metabolism.

8. Minerals
- **Selenium**: Moderate (~20-30µg)
  - Acts as an antioxidant, supporting immune health.
- **Phosphorus**: High (~200-250mg)
  - Crucial for bone health and energy metabolism.
- **Potassium**: Moderate (~250-300mg)
  - Aids in maintaining fluid balance and regulating blood pressure.
- **Iron**: Present (~1-2mg)
  - Important for oxygen transport in the body.
- **Zinc**: Present (~1.0-1.5mg)
  - Supports immune function and wound healing.

9. Amino Acids Profile (Per 100g)	Non-Essential Amino Acids:
Essential Amino Acids:	• **Non-Essential Amino Acids:**
o **Histidine**: ~0.5g	o **Alanine**: ~0.8g
o **Isoleucine**: ~0.9g	o **Aspartic Acid**: ~1.5g
o **Leucine**: ~1.5g	
o **Lysine**: ~2.0g	o **Glutamic Acid**: ~3.2g
o **Methionine**: ~0.4g	
o **Phenylalanine**: ~0.5g	o **Serine**: ~0.6g
o **Threonine**: ~0.7g	o **Glycine**: ~0.5g
o **Tryptophan**: ~0.2g	o **Proline**: ~0.4g
o **Valine**: ~1.1g	o **Tyrosine**: ~0.3g
o **Arginine**: ~1.3g	o **Cysteine**: ~0.2g

Gawra

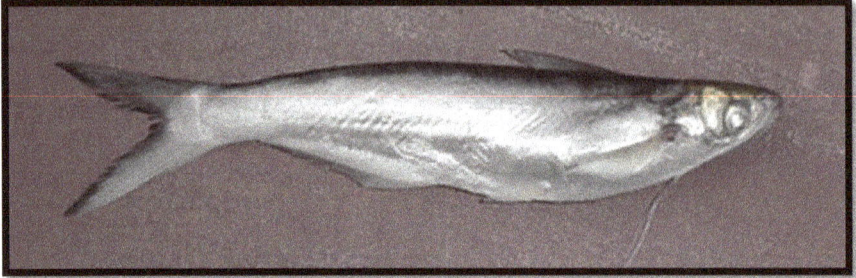

Nutritional Profile of Clupisoma Garua

Common Name: Indian Shad
Scientific Name: Clupisoma garua

1. Oil Content
- **Category**: Medium
- **Oil Breakdown**: Contains about 5-10% total fat, primarily unsaturated fats.

2. Omega Fatty Acids
- **Omega-3**: Approximately 1.5-2.5g per 100g
  - o Supports heart health and reduces inflammation.
- **Omega-6**: Approximately 1.0-2.0g per 100g
  - o Important for cellular function and skin health.
- **Omega-9**: Present in minor amounts.

3. Cholesterol Content
- **Cholesterol**: About 50-70 mg per 100g
  - o Moderate levels, generally acceptable in a balanced diet.

4. Sodium Content
- **Sodium**: Approximately 40-60 mg per 100g
  - o Low sodium, beneficial for managing blood pressure.

5. Mercury Contamination
- **Mercury Levels**: Generally low
  - o Safe for regular consumption, although caution is advised in polluted waters.

6. Nutritional Information (Per 100g)
- **Calories**: ~130 kcal

- **Protein**: ~20-25g
  - High protein content supports muscle growth and repair.
- **Fat**: ~5-10g
  - **Saturated Fat**: ~1.0g
  - **Monounsaturated Fat**: ~2.5g
  - **Polyunsaturated Fat**: ~2.5g

7. Vitamins
- **Vitamin B12**: Present (~2-4μg)
  - Essential for nerve function and red blood cell production.
- **Vitamin D**: Moderate (~40-80 IU)
  - Supports calcium absorption and bone health.
- **Vitamin B6**: Present (~0.3-0.5mg)
  - Important for amino acid metabolism.

8. Minerals
- **Selenium**: Moderate (~15-25μg)
  - Acts as an antioxidant, supporting immune health.
- **Phosphorus**: High (~200-250mg)
  - Crucial for bone health and energy metabolism.
- **Potassium**: Moderate (~300-400mg)
  - Aids in maintaining fluid balance and regulating blood pressure.
- **Iron**: Present (~0.6-1.0mg)
  - Important for oxygen transport in the body.
- **Zinc**: Present (~0.3-0.5mg)
  - Supports immune function and wound healing.

9. Amino Acids Profile (Per 100g) • **Essential Amino Acids**:	• **Non-Essential Amino Acids**:
○ **Histidine**: ~0.9g	○ **Alanine**: ~1.0g
○ **Isoleucine**: ~1.1g	○ **Aspartic Acid**: ~2.2g
○ **Leucine**: ~1.8g	○ **Glutamic Acid**: ~3.0g
○ **Lysine**: ~2.4g	○ **Serine**: ~0.9g
○ **Methionine**: ~0.5g	○ **Glycine**: ~0.6g
○ **Phenylalanine**: ~1.0g	○ **Proline**: ~0.4g
○ **Threonine**: ~0.8g	○ **Tyrosine**: ~0.3g
○ **Tryptophan**: ~0.2g	○ **Cysteine**: ~0.2g
○ **Valine**: ~1.3g	
○ **Arginine**: ~1.5g	

Gonia

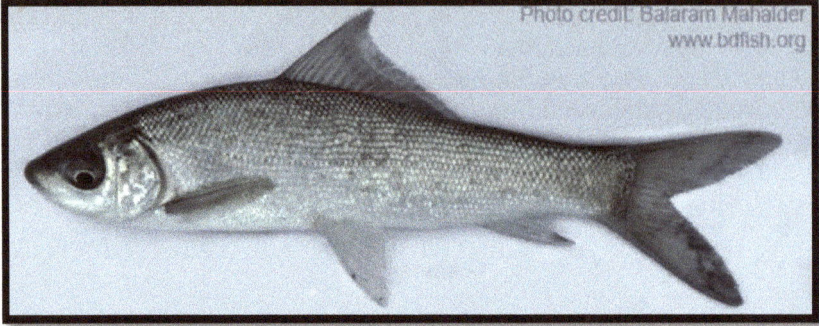

Photo credit: Balaram Mahalder
www.bdfish.org

Nutritional Profile of Kuria Labeo

Common Name: Kuria Fish   **Scientific Name**: Kuria labeo

1. Oil Content
- **Category**: Medium
- **Oil Breakdown**: Contains about 5-10% total fat, primarily unsaturated fats.

2. Omega Fatty Acids
- **Omega-3**: Approximately 1.0-2.0g per 100g
  - Supports heart health and reduces inflammation.
- **Omega-6**: Approximately 1.5-2.5g per 100g
  - Important for cellular function and skin health.
- **Omega-9**: Present in minor amounts.

3. Cholesterol Content
- **Cholesterol**: About 50-70 mg per 100g
  - Moderate levels, generally acceptable in a balanced diet.

4. Sodium Content
- **Sodium**: Approximately 40-60 mg per 100g
  - Low sodium, beneficial for managing blood pressure.

5. Mercury Contamination
- **Mercury Levels**: Generally low
  - Safe for regular consumption, though caution is advised in polluted waters.

6. Nutritional Information (Per 100g)
- **Calories**: ~120 kcal
- **Protein**: ~20-25g
  - High protein content supports muscle growth and repair.
- **Fat**: ~5-10g
  - **Saturated Fat**: ~1.0g
  - **Monounsaturated Fat**: ~2.5g
  - **Polyunsaturated Fat**: ~2.5g

7. Vitamins
- **Vitamin B12**: Present (~2-4µg)
  - Essential for nerve function and red blood cell production.
- **Vitamin D**: Moderate (~50-100 IU)
  - Supports calcium absorption and bone health.
- **Vitamin B6**: Present (~0.3-0.5mg)
  - Important for amino acid metabolism.

8. Minerals
- **Selenium**: Moderate (~15-25µg)
  - Acts as an antioxidant, supporting immune health.
- **Phosphorus**: High (~200-300mg)
  - Crucial for bone health and energy metabolism.
- **Potassium**: Moderate (~300-400mg)
  - Aids in maintaining fluid balance and regulating blood pressure.
- **Iron**: Present (~0.5-1.0mg)
  - Important for oxygen transport in the body.
- **Zinc**: Present (~0.3-0.5mg)
  - Supports immune function and wound healing.

9. Amino Acids Profile (Per 100g)	• Non-Essential Amino
• **Essential Amino Acids:**	**Acids:**
○ **Histidine**: ~0.8g	○ **Alanine**: ~1.0g
○ **Isoleucine**: ~1.1g	○ **Aspartic Acid**: ~2.1g
○ **Leucine**: ~1.7g	○ **Glutamic Acid**: ~3.0g
○ **Lysine**: ~2.3g	○ **Serine**: ~0.9g
○ **Methionine**: ~0.5g	○ **Glycine**: ~0.6g
○ **Phenylalanine**: ~1.0g	○ **Proline**: ~0.4g
○ **Threonine**: ~0.9g	○ **Tyrosine**: ~0.3g
○ **Tryptophan**: ~0.2g	○ **Cysteine**: ~0.2g
○ **Valine**: ~1.3g	
○ **Arginine**: ~1.5g	

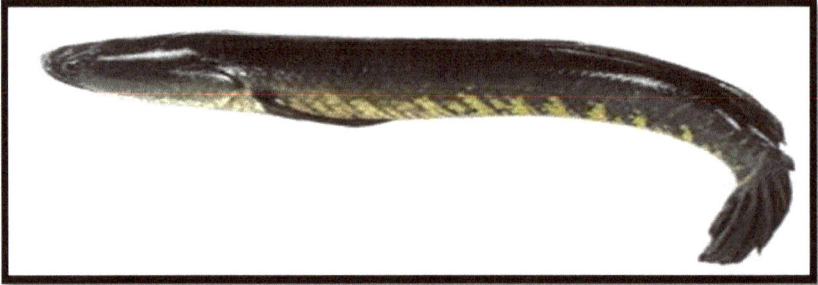

Gozar

Nutritional Profile of Channa Marulius

Common Name: Giant Snakehead, Hole, Shoil
Scientific Name: Channa marulius

1. Oil Content
- **Category**: Fatty
- **Oil Breakdown**: Contains about 10-15% total fat, with a good proportion of unsaturated fats.

2. Omega Fatty Acids
- **Omega-3**: Approximately 1.0-2.0g per 100g
  - Supports cardiovascular health and has anti-inflammatory properties.
- **Omega-6**: Approximately 1.5-2.5g per 100g
  - Important for cellular function and skin health.
- **Omega-9**: Present in minor amounts.

3. Cholesterol Content
- **Cholesterol**: About 60-90 mg per 100g
  - Moderate levels, generally acceptable in a balanced diet.

4. Sodium Content
- **Sodium**: Approximately 50-70 mg per 100g
  - Low sodium, beneficial for managing blood pressure.

5. Mercury Contamination
- **Mercury Levels**: Generally low
  - Safe for regular consumption, though caution is advised in polluted waters.

6. Nutritional Information (Per 100g)

- **Calories**: ~130 kcal
- **Protein**: ~20-25g
    - High protein content supports muscle growth and repair.
- **Fat**: ~10-15g
    - **Saturated Fat**: ~2.5g
    - **Monounsaturated Fat**: ~5.0g
    - **Polyunsaturated Fat**: ~3.0g

7. Vitamins

- **Vitamin B12**: Present (~3-5µg)
    - Essential for nerve function and red blood cell production.
- **Vitamin D**: Moderate (~50-100 IU)
    - Supports calcium absorption and bone health.
- **Vitamin B6**: Present (~0.3-0.5mg)
    - Important for amino acid metabolism.

8. Minerals

- **Selenium**: Moderate (~20-30µg)
    - Acts as an antioxidant, supporting immune health.
- **Phosphorus**: High (~200-300mg)
    - Crucial for bone health and energy metabolism.
- **Potassium**: Moderate (~300-400mg)
    - Aids in maintaining fluid balance and regulating blood pressure.
- **Iron**: Present (~0.6-1.0mg)
    - Important for oxygen transport in the body.
- **Zinc**: Present (~0.4-0.6mg)
    - Supports immune function and wound healing.

9. Amino Acids Profile (Per 100g)	• Non-Essential Amino Acids:
• **Essential Amino Acids**:	
○ **Histidine**: ~0.8g	○ **Alanine**: ~1.2g
○ **Isoleucine**: ~1.2g	○ **Aspartic Acid**: ~2.3g
○ **Leucine**: ~1.7g	
○ **Lysine**: ~2.5g	○ **Glutamic Acid**: ~3.5g
○ **Methionine**: ~0.5g	
○ **Phenylalanine**: ~1.1g	○ **Serine**: ~1.0g
○ **Threonine**: ~0.9g	○ **Glycine**: ~0.8g
○ **Tryptophan**: ~0.3g	○ **Proline**: ~0.5g
○ **Valine**: ~1.5g	○ **Tyrosine**: ~0.4g
○ **Arginine**: ~1.6g	○ **Cysteine**: ~0.3g

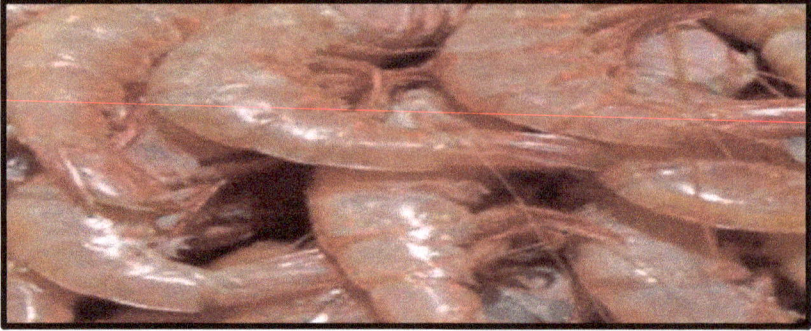

Harina

Nutritional Profile of Metapenaeus monoceros

Common Name: White Shrimp
Scientific Name: Metapenaeus monoceros

1. Oil Content
- **Category**: Lean to medium-fat
- **Oil Breakdown**: Approximately 1-3% total fat, primarily unsaturated fats.

2. Omega Fatty Acids
- **Omega-3**: About 0.2-0.5g per 100g
    o   Supports heart health and reduces inflammation.
- **Omega-6**: Approximately 0.5-1.0g per 100g
    o   Important for skin health and cellular functions.
- **Omega-9**: Present in small amounts.

3. Cholesterol Content
- **Cholesterol**: About 150-200 mg per 100g
    o   Higher levels; should be consumed in moderation.

4. Sodium Content
- **Sodium**: Approximately 500-800 mg per 100g
    o   Higher sodium content; consider for blood pressure management.

5. Mercury Contamination
- **Mercury Levels**: Low to moderate
    o   Generally safe for consumption but check local advisories.

6. Nutritional Information (Per 100g)
- **Calories**: ~80-90 kcal
- **Protein**: ~15-20g
  - High protein content supports muscle growth and repair.
- **Fat**: ~1-3g
  - **Saturated Fat**: ~0.3-0.5g
  - **Monounsaturated Fat**: ~0.2g
  - **Polyunsaturated Fat**: ~0.3g

7. Vitamins
- **Vitamin B12**: High (~2-4µg)
  - Essential for nerve function and red blood cell production.
- **Vitamin D**: Present (~10-20 IU)
  - Important for bone health and calcium absorption.
- **Vitamin B6**: Low (~0.1-0.2mg)

8. Minerals
- **Selenium**: High (~30-40µg)
  - Acts as an antioxidant, supporting immune health.
- **Phosphorus**: Moderate (~200-250mg)
  - Crucial for bone health and energy metabolism.
- **Potassium**: Moderate (~200-250mg)
  - Aids in maintaining fluid balance and regulating blood pressure.
- **Iron**: Present (~1.0-1.5mg)
  - Important for oxygen transport in the body.

9. Amino Acids Profile (Per 100g)	Non-Essential Amino Acids:
Essential Amino Acids:	o **Alanine**: ~0.5g
o **Histidine**: ~0.6g	o **Aspartic Acid**: ~1.1g
o **Isoleucine**: ~0.9g	o **Glutamic Acid**: ~2.0g
o **Leucine**: ~1.3g	o **Serine**: ~0.4g
o **Lysine**: ~1.6g	o **Glycine**: ~0.5g
o **Methionine**: ~0.5g	o **Proline**: ~0.3g
o **Phenylalanine**: ~0.6g	o **Tyrosine**: ~0.3g
o **Threonine**: ~0.8g	o **Cysteine**: ~0.2g
o **Tryptophan**: ~0.2g	
o **Valine**: ~1.0g	
o **Arginine**: ~1.0g	

Herring

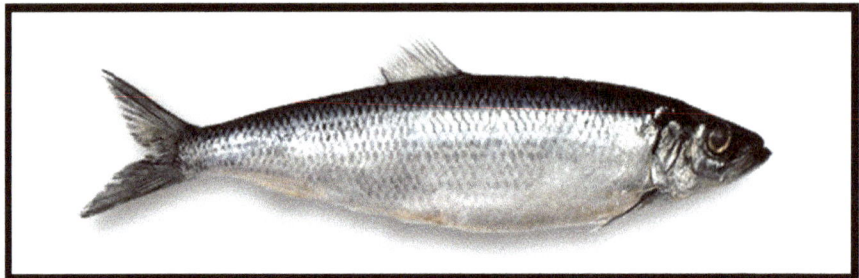

Nutritional Profile of Herring

Common Name: Herring   **Scientific Name**: Clupea harengus

1. Oil Content
- **Category**: Fatty
- **Oil Breakdown**: Contains about 15-25% total fat, predominantly unsaturated fats.

2. Omega Fatty Acids
- **Omega-3**: Approximately 2.0-2.5g per 100g
  - Supports heart health, reduces inflammation, and aids cognitive function.
- **Omega-6**: Approximately 0.5-1.0g per 100g
  - Important for cellular health and metabolism.
- **Omega-9**: Present in smaller amounts.

3. Cholesterol Content
- **Cholesterol**: About 50-60 mg per 100g
  - Moderate levels; generally acceptable in a balanced diet.

4. Sodium Content
- **Sodium**: Approximately 50-70 mg per 100g (may vary with preparation)
  - Low sodium, beneficial for blood pressure management.

5. Mercury Contamination
- **Mercury Levels**: Generally low
  - Safe for regular consumption, though caution is advised with larger fish.

6. Nutritional Information (Per 100g)
- **Calories**: ~200 kcal
- **Protein**: ~20-25g
  - High protein content supports muscle growth and repair.
- **Fat**: ~15-25g
  - **Saturated Fat**: ~2-3g
  - **Monounsaturated Fat**: ~4-6g
  - **Polyunsaturated Fat**: ~8-15g

7. Vitamins
- **Vitamin B12**: High (~12-15µg)
  - Essential for nerve function and red blood cell production.
- **Vitamin D**: High (~600-800 IU)
  - Supports calcium absorption and bone health.
- **Vitamin B6**: Moderate (~0.5-1.0mg)
  - Important for amino acid metabolism.

8. Minerals
- **Selenium**: High (~30-40µg)
  - Acts as an antioxidant, supporting immune health.
- **Phosphorus**: Moderate (~200-250mg)
  - Crucial for bone health and energy metabolism.
- **Potassium**: Moderate (~300-400mg)
  - Aids in fluid balance and blood pressure regulation.
- **Iron**: Present (~1.0-1.5mg)
  - Important for oxygen transport in the body.
- **Zinc**: Present (~0.5-1.0mg)
  - Supports immune function and wound healing.

9. Amino Acids Profile (Per 100g)	• Non-Essential Amino
• **Essential Amino Acids**:	Acids:
○ **Histidine**: ~1.0g	○ **Alanine**: ~1.1g
○ **Isoleucine**: ~1.2g	○ **Aspartic Acid**: ~2.5g
○ **Leucine**: ~1.8g	○ **Glutamic Acid**: ~3.5g
○ **Lysine**: ~2.5g	○ **Serine**: ~1.0g
○ **Methionine**: ~0.6g	○ **Glycine**: ~0.7g
○ **Phenylalanine**: ~1.1g	○ **Proline**: ~0.5g
○ **Threonine**: ~0.9g	○ **Tyrosine**: ~0.4g
○ **Tryptophan**: ~0.3g	○ **Cysteine**: ~0.3g
○ **Valine**: ~1.5g	
○ **Arginine**: ~1.5g	

Hichiri Moila

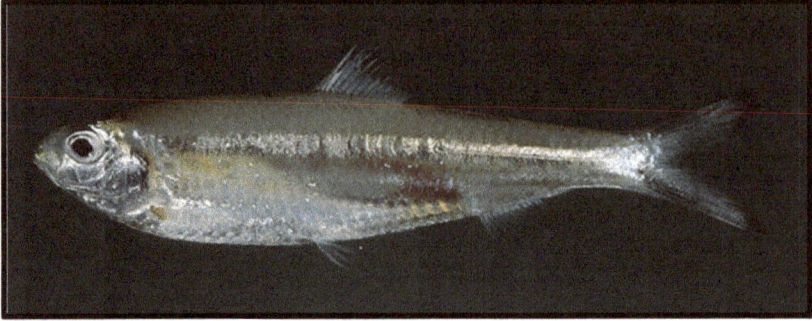

Nutritional Profile of Escualosa thoracata

Common Name: Hichiri Moila
Scientific Name: Escualosa thoracata

1. Oil Content
- **Category**: Fatty
- **Oil Breakdown**: Approximately 10-15% total fat, primarily unsaturated fats.

2. Omega Fatty Acids
- **Omega-3**: About 1.0-2.0g per 100g
  - Supports heart health and reduces inflammation.
- **Omega-6**: Approximately 0.5-1.0g per 100g
  - Important for skin health and cellular functions.
- **Omega-9**: Present in moderate amounts.

3. Cholesterol Content
- **Cholesterol**: About 60-80 mg per 100g
  - Moderate levels; generally acceptable for most diets.

4. Sodium Content
- **Sodium**: Approximately 50-70 mg per 100g
  - Moderate sodium content; beneficial for blood pressure management.

5. Mercury Contamination
- **Mercury Levels**: Low
  - Generally safe for consumption with minimal risk of mercury contamination.

6. Nutritional Information (Per 100g)
- **Calories**: ~130-150 kcal
- **Protein**: ~20-25g
  - High protein content supports muscle growth and repair.
- **Fat**: ~10-15g
  - **Saturated Fat**: ~2.0-3.0g
  - **Monounsaturated Fat**: ~3.0-4.0g
  - **Polyunsaturated Fat**: ~5.0-6.0g

7. Vitamins
- **Vitamin B12**: High (~2-4µg)
  - Essential for nerve function and red blood cell production.
- **Vitamin D**: Moderate (~10-20 IU)
  - Important for bone health and calcium absorption.
- **Vitamin B6**: Present (~0.5-0.7mg)
  - Important for amino acid metabolism.

8. Minerals
- **Selenium**: High (~25-35µg)
  - Acts as an antioxidant, supporting immune health.
- **Phosphorus**: Moderate (~200-250mg)
  - Crucial for bone health and energy metabolism.
- **Potassium**: Moderate (~200-250mg)
  - Aids in maintaining fluid balance and regulating blood pressure.
- **Iron**: Present (~0.7-1.0mg)
  - Important for oxygen transport in the body.

9. Amino Acids Profile (Per 100g)	Non-Essential Amino Acids:
Essential Amino Acids:	
Histidine: ~0.4g	Alanine: ~0.6g
Isoleucine: ~1.0g	Aspartic Acid: ~1.3g
Leucine: ~1.5g	Glutamic Acid: ~2.2g
Lysine: ~1.6g	Serine: ~0.5g
Methionine: ~0.4g	Glycine: ~0.5g
Phenylalanine: ~0.7g	Proline: ~0.4g
Threonine: ~0.8g	Tyrosine: ~0.3g
Tryptophan: ~0.2g	Cysteine: ~0.2g
Valine: ~1.0g	
Arginine: ~0.9g	

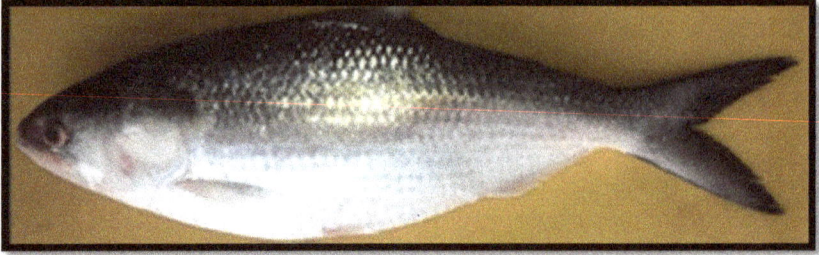

Hilsha

Nutritional Profile of Tenualosa Ilish

Common Name: Hilsa Herring   **Scientific Name**: Tenualosa ilisha

1. Oil Content
- **Category**: Fatty
- **Oil Breakdown**: Contains about 15-20% total fat, primarily unsaturated fats.

2. Omega Fatty Acids
- **Omega-3**: Approximately 2.0-3.5g per 100g
  - o   Supports heart health, reduces inflammation, and promotes brain function.
- **Omega-6**: Approximately 1.0-2.0g per 100g
  - o   Important for cellular health and skin integrity.
- **Omega-9**: Present in smaller amounts.

3. Cholesterol Content
- **Cholesterol**: About 70-90 mg per 100g
  - o   Moderate levels, generally acceptable within a balanced diet.

4. Sodium Content
- **Sodium**: Approximately 50-70 mg per 100g
  - o   Low sodium, beneficial for managing blood pressure.

5. Mercury Contamination
- **Mercury Levels**: Generally low
  - o   Safe for regular consumption, though caution is advised in polluted waters.

6. Nutritional Information (Per 100g)
- **Calories**: ~200 kcal

- **Protein**: ~20-25g
  - High protein content supports muscle growth and repair.
- **Fat**: ~15-20g
  - **Saturated Fat**: ~2-3g
  - **Monounsaturated Fat**: ~5-7g
  - **Polyunsaturated Fat**: ~8-10g

7. Vitamins
- **Vitamin B12**: High (~10-15µg)
  - Essential for nerve function and red blood cell production.
- **Vitamin D**: Moderate (~300-500 IU)
  - Supports calcium absorption and bone health.
- **Vitamin B6**: Present (~0.5-1.0mg)
  - Important for amino acid metabolism.

8. Minerals
- **Selenium**: High (~30-40µg)
  - Acts as an antioxidant, supporting immune health.
- **Phosphorus**: High (~200-250mg)
  - Crucial for bone health and energy metabolism.
- **Potassium**: Moderate (~300-400mg)
  - Aids in maintaining fluid balance and regulating blood pressure.
- **Iron**: Present (~1.0-1.5mg)
  - Important for oxygen transport in the body.
- **Zinc**: Present (~0.4-0.8mg)
  - Supports immune function and wound healing.

9. Amino Acids Profile (Per 100g)	Non-Essential Amino Acids:
Essential Amino Acids:	• **Non-Essential Amino Acids:**
o **Histidine**: ~1.0g	o **Alanine**: ~1.2g
o **Isoleucine**: ~1.3g	o **Aspartic Acid**: ~2.4g
o **Leucine**: ~1.9g	o **Glutamic Acid**: ~3.6g
o **Lysine**: ~2.4g	o **Serine**: ~1.1g
o **Methionine**: ~0.5g	o **Glycine**: ~0.8g
o **Phenylalanine**: ~1.1g	o **Proline**: ~0.5g
o **Threonine**: ~0.9g	o **Tyrosine**: ~0.4g
o **Tryptophan**: ~0.3g	o **Cysteine**: ~0.3g
o **Valine**: ~1.4g	
o **Arginine**: ~1.5g	

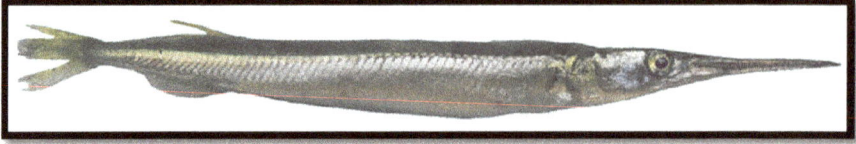

Kakila

Nutritional Profile of Xenentodon Cancila

Common Name: Freshwater Needlefish
Scientific Name: Xenentodon cancila

1. Oil Content
- **Category**: Lean
- **Oil Breakdown**: Contains about 4-8% total fat, mostly unsaturated fats.

2. Omega Fatty Acids
- **Omega-3**: Approximately 0.5-1.0g per 100g
  - Supports cardiovascular health and reduces inflammation.
- **Omega-6**: Approximately 0.3-0.6g per 100g
  - Important for cell structure and overall health.
- **Omega-9**: Present in smaller amounts.

3. Cholesterol Content
- **Cholesterol**: About 30-40 mg per 100g
  - Low levels, suitable for a healthy diet.

4. Sodium Content
- **Sodium**: Approximately 40-60 mg per 100g
  - Low sodium, beneficial for blood pressure management.

5. Mercury Contamination
- **Mercury Levels**: Generally low
  - Safe for regular consumption, though monitoring is advised in polluted waters.

6. Nutritional Information (Per 100g)
- **Calories**: ~120 kcal
- **Protein**: ~20-22g
  - High protein content supports muscle growth and repair.
- **Fat**: ~4-8g
  - **Saturated Fat**: ~1g

- o **Monounsaturated Fat**: ~1-2g
- o **Polyunsaturated Fat**: ~2-5g

7. Vitamins

- **Vitamin B12**: Moderate (~2-3µg)
  - o Essential for nerve function and red blood cell production.
- **Vitamin D**: Present (~100-200 IU)
  - o Supports calcium absorption and bone health.
- **Vitamin B6**: Low (~0.2-0.4mg)
  - o Important for amino acid metabolism.

8. Minerals

- **Selenium**: Moderate (~15-20µg)
  - o Acts as an antioxidant, supporting immune health.
- **Phosphorus**: Moderate (~150-200mg)
  - o Crucial for bone health and energy metabolism.
- **Potassium**: Moderate (~250-350mg)
  - o Aids in maintaining fluid balance and regulating blood pressure.
- **Iron**: Present (~0.5-1.0mg)
  - o Important for oxygen transport in the body.
- **Zinc**: Present (~0.4-0.6mg)
  - o Supports immune function and wound healing.

9. Amino Acids Profile (Per 100g)	• Non-Essential Amino Acids:
• **Essential Amino Acids:**	o **Alanine**: ~1.0g
o **Histidine**: ~0.7g	o **Aspartic Acid**: ~2.0g
o **Isoleucine**: ~1.0g	o **Glutamic Acid**: ~3.0g
o **Leucine**: ~1.5g	o **Serine**: ~0.9g
o **Lysine**: ~2.0g	o **Glycine**: ~0.6g
o **Methionine**: ~0.4g	o **Proline**: ~0.4g
o **Phenylalanine**: ~0.9g	o **Tyrosine**: ~0.3g
o **Threonine**: ~0.8g	o **Cysteine**: ~0.2g
o **Tryptophan**: ~0.2g	
o **Valine**: ~1.2g	
o **Arginine**: ~1.3g	

Kali Bawsh

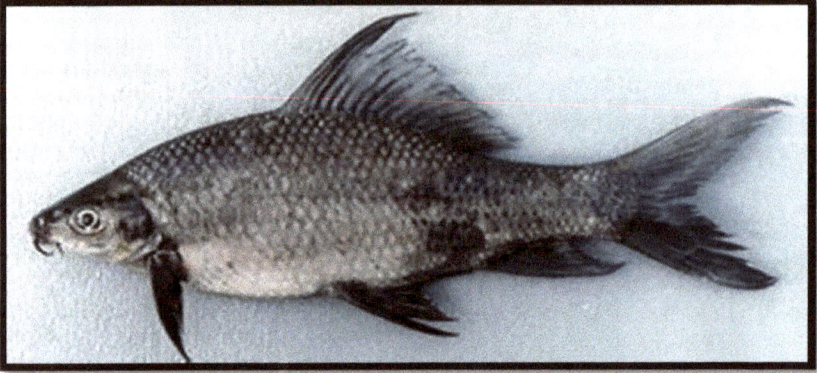

Nutritional Profile of Labeo Calbasu

Common Name: Indian Carp   **Scientific Name**: Labeo calbasu

1. Oil Content
- **Category**: Medium
- **Oil Breakdown**: Contains about 5-10% total fat, primarily unsaturated fats.

2. Omega Fatty Acids
- **Omega-3**: Approximately 0.5-1.0g per 100g
  - Supports heart health and reduces inflammation.
- **Omega-6**: Approximately 1.0-1.5g per 100g
  - Important for cellular functions and skin health.
- **Omega-9**: Present in smaller amounts.

3. Cholesterol Content
- **Cholesterol**: About 40-60 mg per 100g
  - Moderate levels, generally acceptable in a healthy diet.

4. Sodium Content
- **Sodium**: Approximately 50-70 mg per 100g
  - Low sodium, beneficial for blood pressure management.

5. Mercury Contamination
- **Mercury Levels**: Generally low
  - Safe for regular consumption, though monitoring is advised in polluted waters.

6. Nutritional Information (Per 100g)
- **Calories**: ~130 kcal
- **Protein**: ~18-20g
  - High protein content supports muscle growth and repair.
- **Fat**: ~5-10g
  - **Saturated Fat**: ~1-2g
  - **Monounsaturated Fat**: ~2-3g
  - **Polyunsaturated Fat**: ~2-5g

7. Vitamins
- **Vitamin B12**: Moderate (~2-3µg)
  - Essential for nerve function and red blood cell production.
- **Vitamin D**: Low (~50-100 IU)
  - Supports calcium absorption and bone health.
- **Vitamin B6**: Present (~0.3-0.5mg)
  - Important for amino acid metabolism.

8. Minerals
- **Selenium**: Moderate (~20-25µg)
  - Acts as an antioxidant, supporting immune health.
- **Phosphorus**: Moderate (~150-200mg)
  - Crucial for bone health and energy metabolism.
- **Potassium**: Moderate (~300-400mg)
  - Aids in maintaining fluid balance and regulating blood pressure.
- **Iron**: Present (~0.5-1.0mg)
  - Important for oxygen transport in the body.
- **Zinc**: Present (~0.4-0.8mg)
  - Supports immune function and wound healing.

9. Amino Acids Profile (Per 100g)	Non-Essential Amino Acids:
Essential Amino Acids: o **Histidine**: ~0.8g o **Isoleucine**: ~1.1g o **Leucine**: ~1.6g o **Lysine**: ~2.0g o **Methionine**: ~0.4g o **Phenylalanine**: ~0.8g o **Threonine**: ~0.7g o **Tryptophan**: ~0.3g o **Valine**: ~1.3g o **Arginine**: ~1.4g	o **Alanine**: ~1.1g o **Aspartic Acid**: ~2.2g o **Glutamic Acid**: ~3.4g o **Serine**: ~0.8g o **Glycine**: ~0.7g o **Proline**: ~0.5g o **Tyrosine**: ~0.4g o **Cysteine**: ~0.3g

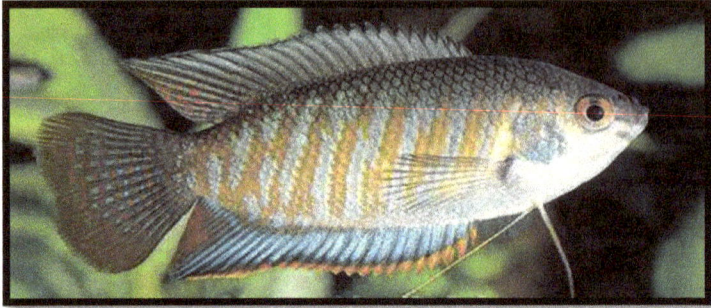

Kalisha

Nutritional Profile of Colisa Fasciatus

Common Name: Zebra Fish   **Scientific Name**: Colisa fasciatus

1. Oil Content
- **Category**: Lean
- **Oil Breakdown**: Contains about 3-5% total fat, primarily unsaturated fats.

2. Omega Fatty Acids
- **Omega-3**: Approximately 0.3-0.5g per 100g
  - o Supports cardiovascular health and reduces inflammation.
- **Omega-6**: Approximately 0.5-1.0g per 100g
  - o Important for skin health and cellular function.
- **Omega-9**: Present in smaller amounts.

3. Cholesterol Content
- **Cholesterol**: About 25-35 mg per 100g
  - o Low levels, suitable for a healthy diet.

4. Sodium Content
- **Sodium**: Approximately 40-60 mg per 100g
  - o Low sodium, beneficial for blood pressure management.

5. Mercury Contamination
- **Mercury Levels**: Generally low
  - o Safe for regular consumption, though monitoring is advised in polluted waters.

6. Nutritional Information (Per 100g)
- **Calories**: ~100 kcal

- **Protein**: ~16-18g
  - High protein content supports muscle growth and repair.
- **Fat**: ~3-5g
  - **Saturated Fat**: ~0.5g
  - **Monounsaturated Fat**: ~1-2g
  - **Polyunsaturated Fat**: ~1-2g

7. Vitamins

- **Vitamin B12**: Moderate (~1-2µg)
  - Essential for nerve function and red blood cell production.
- **Vitamin D**: Low (~20-50 IU)
  - Supports calcium absorption and bone health.
- **Vitamin B6**: Present (~0.2-0.4mg)
  - Important for amino acid metabolism.

8. Minerals

- **Selenium**: Moderate (~15-20µg)
  - Acts as an antioxidant, supporting immune health.
- **Phosphorus**: Moderate (~120-150mg)
  - Crucial for bone health and energy metabolism.
- **Potassium**: Moderate (~250-300mg)
  - Aids in maintaining fluid balance and regulating blood pressure.
- **Iron**: Present (~0.5-1.0mg)
  - Important for oxygen transport in the body.
- **Zinc**: Present (~0.3-0.6mg)
  - Supports immune function and wound healing.

9. Amino Acids Profile (Per 100g)	• Non-Essential Amino
• Essential Amino Acids:	Acids:
○ **Histidine**: ~0.6g	○ **Alanine**: ~1.0g
○ **Isoleucine**: ~1.0g	○ **Aspartic Acid**: ~2.0g
○ **Leucine**: ~1.5g	○ **Glutamic Acid**: ~3.0g
○ **Lysine**: ~1.8g	○ **Serine**: ~0.8g
○ **Methionine**: ~0.3g	○ **Glycine**: ~0.5g
○ **Phenylalanine**: ~0.7g	○ **Proline**: ~0.4g
○ **Threonine**: ~0.7g	○ **Tyrosine**: ~0.3g
○ **Tryptophan**: ~0.2g	○ **Cysteine**: ~0.2g
○ **Valine**: ~1.2g	
○ **Arginine**: ~1.0g	

Katla

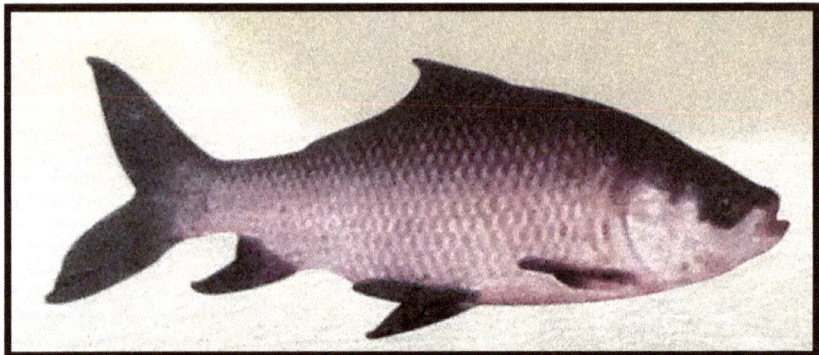

Nutritional Profile of Catla Catla

Common Name: Catla Fish   **Scientific Name**: Catla catla

1. Oil Content
- **Category**: Fatty
- **Oil Breakdown**: Contains about 10-15% total fat, primarily unsaturated fats.

2. Omega Fatty Acids
- **Omega-3**: Approximately 1.0-1.5g per 100g
  - o Supports heart health and reduces inflammation.
- **Omega-6**: Approximately 2.0-3.0g per 100g
  - o Important for skin health and cellular functions.
- **Omega-9**: Present in moderate amounts.

3. Cholesterol Content
- **Cholesterol**: About 50-70 mg per 100g
  - o Relatively low levels, suitable for a healthy diet.

4. Sodium Content
- **Sodium**: Approximately 60-80 mg per 100g
  - o Moderate sodium content; mindful consumption is recommended.

5. Mercury Contamination
- **Mercury Levels**: Generally low
  - o Safe for regular consumption, though care should be taken in polluted waters.

6. Nutritional Information (Per 100g)
- Calories: ~120-150 kcal
- Protein: ~18-20g
    - High protein content supports muscle growth and repair.
- Fat: ~10-15g
    - Saturated Fat: ~2-4g
    - Monounsaturated Fat: ~4-6g
    - Polyunsaturated Fat: ~4-6g

7. Vitamins
- Vitamin B12: High (~3-5µg)
    - Essential for nerve function and red blood cell production.
- Vitamin D: Moderate (~100-200 IU)
    - Supports calcium absorption and bone health.
- Vitamin B6: Present (~0.5-0.8mg)
    - Important for amino acid metabolism.

8. Minerals
- Selenium: Moderate (~20-30µg)
    - Acts as an antioxidant, supporting immune health.
- Phosphorus: High (~200-250mg)
    - Crucial for bone health and energy metabolism.
- Potassium: Moderate (~300-350mg)
    - Aids in maintaining fluid balance and regulating blood pressure.
- Iron: Present (~0.6-1.0mg)
    - Important for oxygen transport in the body.
- Zinc: Present (~0.5-0.8mg)
    - Supports immune function and wound healing.

9. Amino Acids Profile (Per 100g)	Non-Essential Amino Acids:
Essential Amino Acids:	
Histidine: ~0.6g	Alanine: ~1.0g
Isoleucine: ~1.2g	Aspartic Acid: ~2.0g
Leucine: ~1.8g	Glutamic Acid: ~4.0g
Lysine: ~2.0g	Serine: ~0.8g
Methionine: ~0.4g	Glycine: ~0.6g
Phenylalanine: ~0.8g	Proline: ~0.4g
Threonine: ~1.0g	Tyrosine: ~0.3g
Tryptophan: ~0.3g	Cysteine: ~0.2g
Valine: ~1.3g	
Arginine: ~1.0g	

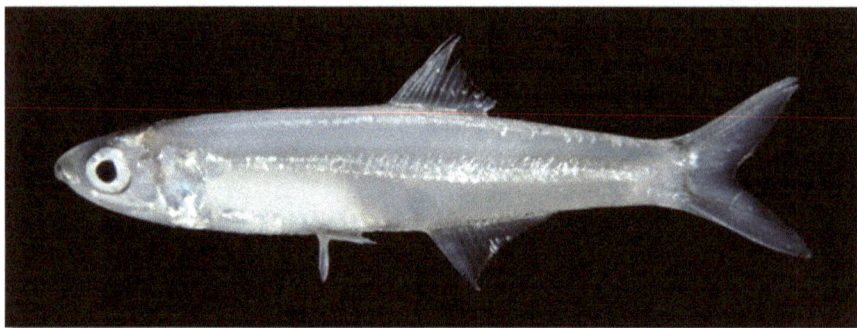

Keski (Anchovy (devil)

Nutritional Profile of Stolephorus Commersonii

Common Name: Indian Anchovy
Scientific Name: Stolephorus commersonii

1. Oil Content
- **Category**: Fatty
- **Oil Breakdown**: Contains about 15-25% total fat, rich in unsaturated fats.

2. Omega Fatty Acids
- **Omega-3**: Approximately 1.5-2.5g per 100g
    - Supports cardiovascular health and reduces inflammation.
- **Omega-6**: Approximately 1.0-2.0g per 100g
    - Important for skin health and cellular functions.
- **Omega-9**: Present in moderate amounts.

3. Cholesterol Content
- **Cholesterol**: About 40-60 mg per 100g
    - Relatively low levels, suitable for a healthy diet.

4. Sodium Content
- **Sodium**: Approximately 60-80 mg per 100g
    - Moderate sodium content; mindful consumption is recommended.

5. Mercury Contamination
- **Mercury Levels**: Generally low
    - Safe for regular consumption, though care should be taken in polluted waters.

6. Nutritional Information (Per 100g)

- **Calories**: ~180 kcal
- **Protein**: ~20-22g
  - High protein content supports muscle growth and repair.
- **Fat**: ~15-25g
  - **Saturated Fat**: ~3-5g
  - **Monounsaturated Fat**: ~5-10g
  - **Polyunsaturated Fat**: ~7-12g

7. Vitamins

- **Vitamin B12**: High (~10-15µg)
  - Essential for nerve function and red blood cell production.
- **Vitamin D**: Moderate (~200-300 IU)
  - Supports calcium absorption and bone health.
- **Vitamin B6**: Present (~0.5-1.0mg)
  - Important for amino acid metabolism.

8. Minerals

- **Selenium**: Moderate (~30-40µg)
  - Acts as an antioxidant, supporting immune health.
- **Phosphorus**: High (~250-300mg)
  - Crucial for bone health and energy metabolism.
- **Potassium**: Moderate (~300-400mg)
  - Aids in maintaining fluid balance and regulating blood pressure.
- **Iron**: Present (~1.0-1.5mg)
  - Important for oxygen transport in the body.
- **Zinc**: Present (~0.8-1.0mg)
  - Supports immune function and wound healing.

9. Amino Acids Profile (Per 100g)	Non-Essential Amino Acids:
Essential Amino Acids:	<ul><li>**Alanine**: ~1.2g</li></ul>
<ul><li>**Histidine**: ~1.0g</li><li>**Isoleucine**: ~1.2g</li><li>**Leucine**: ~1.8g</li><li>**Lysine**: ~2.5g</li><li>**Methionine**: ~0.5g</li><li>**Phenylalanine**: ~1.0g</li><li>**Threonine**: ~1.0g</li><li>**Tryptophan**: ~0.3g</li><li>**Valine**: ~1.5g</li><li>**Arginine**: ~1.4g</li></ul>	<ul><li>**Aspartic Acid**: ~2.5g</li><li>**Glutamic Acid**: ~4.0g</li><li>**Serine**: ~1.0g</li><li>**Glycine**: ~0.8g</li><li>**Proline**: ~0.5g</li><li>**Tyrosine**: ~0.4g</li><li>**Cysteine**: ~0.3g</li></ul>

Keski (Anchovy (Spotty-face)

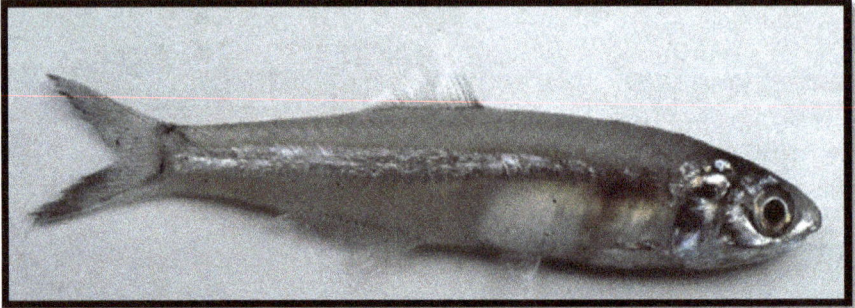

Nutritional Profile of Stolephorus Waitei

Common Name: Indian Anchovy
Scientific Name: Stolephorus waitei

1. Oil Content
- **Category**: Fatty
- **Oil Breakdown**: Contains about 15-25% total fat, primarily unsaturated fats.

2. Omega Fatty Acids
- **Omega-3**: Approximately 1.5-2.5g per 100g
  - Supports heart health and reduces inflammation.
- **Omega-6**: Approximately 1.0-2.0g per 100g
  - Important for skin health and cellular functions.
- **Omega-9**: Present in moderate amounts.

3. Cholesterol Content
- **Cholesterol**: About 50-70 mg per 100g
  - Relatively low levels, suitable for a healthy diet.

4. Sodium Content
- **Sodium**: Approximately 60-90 mg per 100g
  - Moderate sodium content; mindful consumption is recommended.

5. Mercury Contamination
- **Mercury Levels**: Generally low
  - Safe for regular consumption, although care should be taken in polluted waters.

6. Nutritional Information (Per 100g)

- **Calories**: ~180 kcal
- **Protein**: ~20-22g
  - High protein content supports muscle growth and repair.
- **Fat**: ~15-25g
  - **Saturated Fat**: ~3-5g
  - **Monounsaturated Fat**: ~5-10g
  - **Polyunsaturated Fat**: ~7-12g

7. Vitamins

- **Vitamin B12**: High (~10-15μg)
  - Essential for nerve function and red blood cell production.
- **Vitamin D**: Moderate (~200-300 IU)
  - Supports calcium absorption and bone health.
- **Vitamin B6**: Present (~0.5-1.0mg)
  - Important for amino acid metabolism.

8. Minerals

- **Selenium**: Moderate (~30-40μg)
  - Acts as an antioxidant, supporting immune health.
- **Phosphorus**: High (~250-300mg)
  - Crucial for bone health and energy metabolism.
- **Potassium**: Moderate (~300-400mg)
  - Aids in maintaining fluid balance and regulating blood pressure.
- **Iron**: Present (~1.0-1.5mg)
  - Important for oxygen transport in the body.
- **Zinc**: Present (~0.8-1.0mg)
  - Supports immune function and wound healing.

9. Amino Acids Profile (Per 100g)	Non-Essential Amino Acids:
Essential Amino Acids:	• **Non-Essential Amino Acids:**
o **Histidine**: ~1.0g	o **Alanine**: ~1.2g
o **Isoleucine**: ~1.2g	o **Aspartic Acid**: ~2.5g
o **Leucine**: ~1.8g	o **Glutamic Acid**: ~4.0g
o **Lysine**: ~2.5g	o **Serine**: ~1.0g
o **Methionine**: ~0.5g	o **Glycine**: ~0.8g
o **Phenylalanine**: ~1.0g	o **Proline**: ~0.5g
o **Threonine**: ~1.0g	o **Tyrosine**: ~0.4g
o **Tryptophan**: ~0.3g	o **Cysteine**: ~0.3g
o **Valine**: ~1.5g	
o **Arginine**: ~1.4g	

Keski

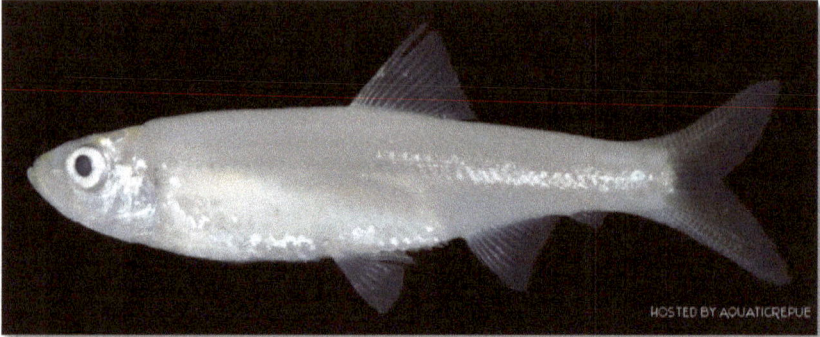

Nutritional Profile of Corica Soborna

Common Name: Keski Fish   **Scientific Name**: Corica soborna

1. Oil Content
- **Category**: Lean
- **Oil Breakdown**: Contains about 3-5% total fat, primarily unsaturated fats.

2. Omega Fatty Acids
- **Omega-3**: Approximately 0.2-0.5g per 100g
  - Supports heart health and reduces inflammation.
- **Omega-6**: Approximately 0.4-0.8g per 100g
  - Important for skin health and cellular functions.
- **Omega-9**: Present in small amounts.

3. Cholesterol Content
- **Cholesterol**: About 30-50 mg per 100g
  - Low levels, suitable for a healthy diet.

4. Sodium Content
- **Sodium**: Approximately 30-60 mg per 100g
  - Low sodium content, beneficial for blood pressure management.

5. Mercury Contamination
- **Mercury Levels**: Generally low
  - Safe for regular consumption, though care should be taken in polluted waters.

6. Nutritional Information (Per 100g)
- **Calories**: ~90-120 kcal
- **Protein**: ~16-18g
  - High protein content supports muscle growth and repair.
- **Fat**: ~3-5g
  - **Saturated Fat**: ~0.5-1g
  - **Monounsaturated Fat**: ~1-2g
  - **Polyunsaturated Fat**: ~1-2g

7. Vitamins
- **Vitamin B12**: Moderate (~2-4µg)
  - Essential for nerve function and red blood cell production.
- **Vitamin D**: Low (~20-40 IU)
  - Supports calcium absorption and bone health.
- **Vitamin B6**: Present (~0.3-0.5mg)
  - Important for amino acid metabolism.

8. Minerals
- **Selenium**: Moderate (~15-25µg)
  - Acts as an antioxidant, supporting immune health.
- **Phosphorus**: Moderate (~150-200mg)
  - Crucial for bone health and energy metabolism.
- **Potassium**: Moderate (~250-350mg)
  - Aids in maintaining fluid balance and regulating blood pressure.
- **Iron**: Present (~0.4-0.6mg)
  - Important for oxygen transport in the body.
- **Zinc**: Present (~0.3-0.5mg)
  - Supports immune function and wound healing.

9. Amino Acids Profile (Per 100g)	**Non-Essential Amino Acids**:
Essential Amino Acids:	○ **Alanine**: ~0.8g
○ **Histidine**: ~0.5g	○ **Aspartic Acid**: ~1.5g
○ **Isoleucine**: ~1.0g	○ **Glutamic Acid**: ~2.0g
○ **Leucine**: ~1.2g	○ **Serine**: ~0.6g
○ **Lysine**: ~1.5g	○ **Glycine**: ~0.4g
○ **Methionine**: ~0.3g	○ **Proline**: ~0.3g
○ **Phenylalanine**: ~0.6g	○ **Tyrosine**: ~0.3g
○ **Threonine**: ~0.6g	○ **Cysteine**: ~0.2g
○ **Tryptophan**: ~0.2g	
○ **Valine**: ~1.0g	
○ **Arginine**: ~0.8g	

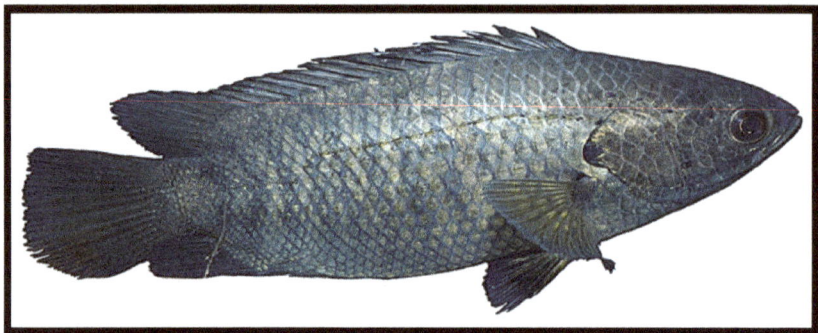

Koi

Nutritional Profile of Anabas Testudineus

Common Name: Climbing Perch
Scientific Name: Anabas testudineus

1. Oil Content
- **Category**: Lean to Moderate
- **Oil Breakdown**: Contains about 5-10% total fat, primarily unsaturated fats.

2. Omega Fatty Acids
- **Omega-3**: Approximately 0.5-1.0g per 100g
   o Supports heart health and reduces inflammation.
- **Omega-6**: Approximately 1.0-2.0g per 100g
   o Important for skin health and cellular functions.
- **Omega-9**: Present in small amounts.

3. Cholesterol Content
- **Cholesterol**: About 40-60 mg per 100g
   o Low cholesterol levels make it suitable for healthy diets.

4. Sodium Content
- **Sodium**: Approximately 40-70 mg per 100g
   o Moderate sodium content; mindful consumption is recommended.

5. Mercury Contamination
- **Mercury Levels**: Generally low
   o Safe for regular consumption, though care should be taken in polluted waters.

6. Nutritional Information (Per 100g)
- **Calories**: ~100-120 kcal
- **Protein**: ~18-20g
  - High protein content supports muscle growth and repair.
- **Fat**: ~5-10g
  - **Saturated Fat**: ~1-2g
  - **Monounsaturated Fat**: ~2-4g
  - **Polyunsaturated Fat**: ~2-3g

7. Vitamins
- **Vitamin B12**: Moderate (~1-3µg)
  - Essential for nerve function and red blood cell production.
- **Vitamin D**: Moderate (~50-100 IU)
  - Supports calcium absorption and bone health.
- **Vitamin B6**: Present (~0.4-0.6mg)
  - Important for amino acid metabolism.

8. Minerals
- **Selenium**: Moderate (~15-25µg)
  - Acts as an antioxidant, supporting immune health.
- **Phosphorus**: High (~200-250mg)
  - Crucial for bone health and energy metabolism.
- **Potassium**: Moderate (~250-350mg)
  - Aids in maintaining fluid balance and regulating blood pressure.
- **Iron**: Present (~0.5-1.0mg)
  - Important for oxygen transport in the body.
- **Zinc**: Present (~0.4-0.6mg)
  - Supports immune function and wound healing.

9. Amino Acids Profile (Per 100g) **Essential Amino Acids:**	**Non-Essential Amino Acids:**
Histidine: ~0.5g	**Alanine**: ~0.9g
Isoleucine: ~1.1g	**Aspartic Acid**: ~1.8g
Leucine: ~1.6g	**Glutamic Acid**: ~3.5g
Lysine: ~1.8g	**Serine**: ~0.6g
Methionine: ~0.3g	**Glycine**: ~0.5g
Phenylalanine: ~0.7g	**Proline**: ~0.4g
Threonine: ~0.7g	**Tyrosine**: ~0.3g
Tryptophan: ~0.3g	**Cysteine**: ~0.2g
Valine: ~1.1g	
Arginine: ~0.9g	

Koral

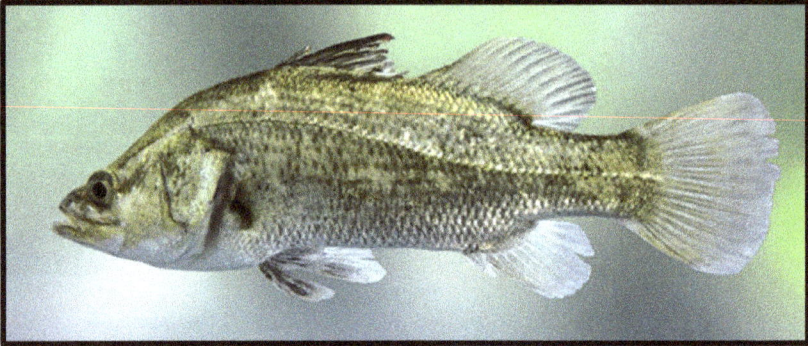

Nutritional Profile of Lates calcarifer

Common Name: Barramundi   **Scientific Name**: Lates calcarifer

1. Oil Content
- **Category**: Fatty
- **Oil Breakdown**: Approximately 10-15% total fat, primarily unsaturated fats.

2. Omega Fatty Acids
- **Omega-3**: About 1.0-1.5g per 100g
  - Supports heart health and reduces inflammation.
- **Omega-6**: Approximately 0.5-1.0g per 100g
  - Important for skin health and cellular functions.
- **Omega-9**: Present in moderate amounts.

3. Cholesterol Content
- **Cholesterol**: About 70-90 mg per 100g
  - Moderate levels; generally acceptable for most diets.

4. Sodium Content
- **Sodium**: Approximately 50-80 mg per 100g
  - Moderate sodium content; consider for blood pressure management.

5. Mercury Contamination
- **Mercury Levels**: Low to moderate
  - Generally safe for consumption but check local advisories.

6. Nutritional Information (Per 100g)

- **Calories**: ~120-150 kcal
- **Protein**: ~20-25g
  - High protein content supports muscle growth and repair.
- **Fat**: ~10-15g
  - **Saturated Fat**: ~3.0-4.0g
  - **Monounsaturated Fat**: ~4.0-5.0g
  - **Polyunsaturated Fat**: ~2.0-3.0g

7. Vitamins

- **Vitamin B12**: High (~3-5μg)
  - Essential for nerve function and red blood cell production.
- **Vitamin D**: High (~20-30 IU)
  - Important for bone health and calcium absorption.
- **Vitamin B6**: Present (~0.5-0.7mg)
  - Important for amino acid metabolism.

8. Minerals

- **Selenium**: High (~30-40μg)
  - Acts as an antioxidant, supporting immune health.
- **Phosphorus**: Moderate (~200-250mg)
  - Crucial for bone health and energy metabolism.
- **Potassium**: Moderate (~250-300mg)
  - Aids in maintaining fluid balance and regulating blood pressure.
- **Iron**: Present (~0.8-1.2mg)
  - Important for oxygen transport in the body.

9. Amino Acids Profile (Per 100g)	Non-Essential Amino Acids:
Essential Amino Acids:	○ **Alanine**: ~0.7g
○ **Histidine**: ~0.5g	○ **Aspartic Acid**: ~1.5g
○ **Isoleucine**: ~1.2g	○ **Glutamic Acid**: ~2.5g
○ **Leucine**: ~1.6g	○ **Serine**: ~0.6g
○ **Lysine**: ~1.8g	○ **Glycine**: ~0.6g
○ **Methionine**: ~0.5g	○ **Proline**: ~0.5g
○ **Phenylalanine**: ~0.8g	○ **Tyrosine**: ~0.4g
○ **Threonine**: ~0.9g	○ **Cysteine**: ~0.3g
○ **Tryptophan**: ~0.2g	
○ **Valine**: ~1.0g	
○ **Arginine**: ~1.0g	

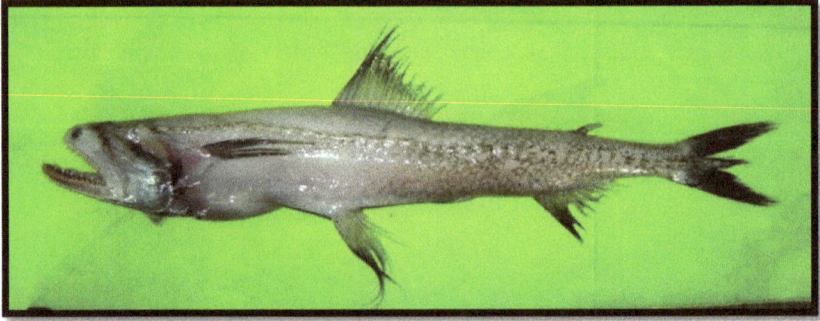

Lohita/Loyta

Nutritional Profile of Harpadon Nehereus

Common Name: Ribbon Fish, Loyta, Bombay Duck
Scientific Name: Harpadon nehereus

1. Oil Content
- **Category**: Fatty
- **Oil Breakdown**: Contains about 10-15% total fat, primarily unsaturated fats.

2. Omega Fatty Acids
- **Omega-3**: Approximately 1.0-2.0g per 100g
  - Supports heart health and reduces inflammation.
- **Omega-6**: Approximately 2.0-3.0g per 100g
  - Important for skin health and cellular functions.
- **Omega-9**: Present in moderate amounts.

3. Cholesterol Content
- **Cholesterol**: About 60-80 mg per 100g
  - Moderate levels; suitable for most diets.

4. Sodium Content
- **Sodium**: Approximately 50-70 mg per 100g
  - Moderate sodium content; mindful consumption is recommended.

5. Mercury Contamination
- **Mercury Levels**: Generally low
  - Safe for regular consumption, though care should be taken in polluted waters.

6. Nutritional Information (Per 100g)
- Calories: ~120-150 kcal
- Protein: ~20-22g
  - High protein content supports muscle growth and repair.
- Fat: ~10-15g
  - **Saturated Fat**: ~2-3g
  - **Monounsaturated Fat**: ~4-6g
  - **Polyunsaturated Fat**: ~4-6g

7. Vitamins
- **Vitamin B12**: High (~2-4µg)
  - Essential for nerve function and red blood cell production.
- **Vitamin D**: Moderate (~100-200 IU)
  - Supports calcium absorption and bone health.
- **Vitamin B6**: Present (~0.5-0.8mg)
  - Important for amino acid metabolism.

8. Minerals
- **Selenium**: Moderate (~20-25µg)
  - Acts as an antioxidant, supporting immune health.
- **Phosphorus**: High (~200-250mg)
  - Crucial for bone health and energy metabolism.
- **Potassium**: Moderate (~300-350mg)
  - Aids in maintaining fluid balance and regulating blood pressure.
- **Iron**: Present (~0.6-1.0mg)
  - Important for oxygen transport in the body.
- **Zinc**: Present (~0.4-0.6mg)
  - Supports immune function and wound healing.

9. Amino Acids Profile (Per 100g)	
Essential Amino Acids:	• **Non-Essential Amino Acids:**
○ **Histidine**: ~0.5g	○ **Alanine**: ~0.9g
○ **Isoleucine**: ~1.2g	○ **Aspartic Acid**: ~2.0g
○ **Leucine**: ~1.8g	○ **Glutamic Acid**: ~4.0g
○ **Lysine**: ~2.1g	○ **Serine**: ~0.7g
○ **Methionine**: ~0.4g	○ **Glycine**: ~0.6g
○ **Phenylalanine**: ~0.7g	○ **Proline**: ~0.5g
○ **Threonine**: ~0.8g	○ **Tyrosine**: ~0.3g
○ **Tryptophan**: ~0.3g	○ **Cysteine**: ~0.2g
○ **Valine**: ~1.3g	
○ **Arginine**: ~1.0g	

Mackerel (Atlantic)

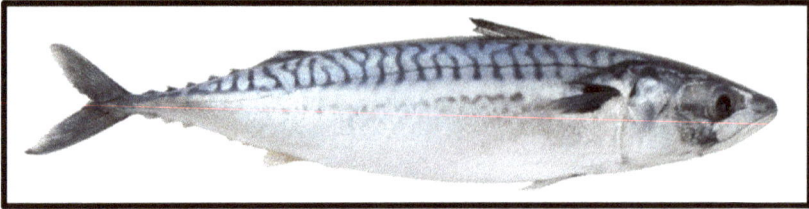

Nutritional Profile of Scomber Scombrus

Common Name: Atlantic Mackerel
Scientific Name: Scomber scombrus

1. Oil Content
- **Category**: Fatty
- **Oil Breakdown**: Contains about 15-25% total fat, primarily unsaturated fats.

2. Omega Fatty Acids
- **Omega-3**: Approximately 2.0-3.5g per 100g
  - o   Supports heart health and reduces inflammation.
- **Omega-6**: Approximately 1.0-2.0g per 100g
  - o   Important for skin health and cellular functions.
- **Omega-9**: Present in moderate amounts.

3. Cholesterol Content
- **Cholesterol**: About 60-80 mg per 100g
  - o   Moderate levels; suitable for most diets.

4. Sodium Content
- **Sodium**: Approximately 50-70 mg per 100g
  - o   Moderate sodium content; mindful consumption is recommended.

5. Mercury Contamination
- **Mercury Levels**: Generally low to moderate
  - o   Safe for regular consumption, though care should be taken in polluted waters.

6. Nutritional Information (Per 100g)
- **Calories**: ~150-200 kcal
- **Protein**: ~20-25g
  - o   High protein content supports muscle growth and repair.

- **Fat**: ~15-25g
  - **Saturated Fat**: ~3-4g
  - **Monounsaturated Fat**: ~6-8g
  - **Polyunsaturated Fat**: ~6-12g

7. Vitamins

- **Vitamin B12**: High (~8-10µg)
  - Essential for nerve function and red blood cell production.
- **Vitamin D**: Moderate (~300-500 IU)
  - Supports calcium absorption and bone health.
- **Vitamin B6**: Present (~0.5-1.0mg)
  - Important for amino acid metabolism.

8. Minerals

- **Selenium**: High (~30-40µg)
  - Acts as an antioxidant, supporting immune health.
- **Phosphorus**: High (~200-250mg)
  - Crucial for bone health and energy metabolism.
- **Potassium**: Moderate (~300-400mg)
  - Aids in maintaining fluid balance and regulating blood pressure.
- **Iron**: Present (~0.5-1.5mg)
  - Important for oxygen transport in the body.
- **Zinc**: Present (~0.5-1.0mg)
  - Supports immune function and wound healing.

9. Amino Acids Profile (Per 100g)	Non-Essential Amino Acids:
Essential Amino Acids: ○ **Histidine**: ~0.5g ○ **Isoleucine**: ~1.3g ○ **Leucine**: ~1.8g ○ **Lysine**: ~2.5g ○ **Methionine**: ~0.5g ○ **Phenylalanine**: ~0.8g ○ **Threonine**: ~0.9g ○ **Tryptophan**: ~0.3g ○ **Valine**: ~1.5g ○ **Arginine**: ~1.1g	○ **Alanine**: ~1.0g ○ **Aspartic Acid**: ~2.5g ○ **Glutamic Acid**: ~4.0g ○ **Serine**: ~0.8g ○ **Glycine**: ~0.7g ○ **Proline**: ~0.5g ○ **Tyrosine**: ~0.4g ○ **Cysteine**: ~0.3g

Safety profile
Scombroid fish poisoning, also known as histamine fish poisoning, is an allergic-type reaction that occurs after consumption of certain improperly refrigerated fish such as tuna, mackerel, amberjack, and bonito. Since histamines are heat-resistant, cooking spoiled fish will not make it safe to eat.
The most common symptoms are rash, diarrhea, reddening of the face and sometimes the neck, arms, and upper part of the body, sweating, headache, palpitations, and vomiting. Urgent medical attention is needed in severe cases.

The Methyl-mercury content of fresh/frozen skipjack tuna is 0.050 PPM, and hence, categorized as the "Best Choice" fish. FDA advises that one can eat 2 to 3 servings a week from the "Best Choice" list (adult 1 serving = 4 ounces). To compare, King mackerel has 0.73 ppm; categorizing it in the list- "avoid".

Mackerel (Indian)

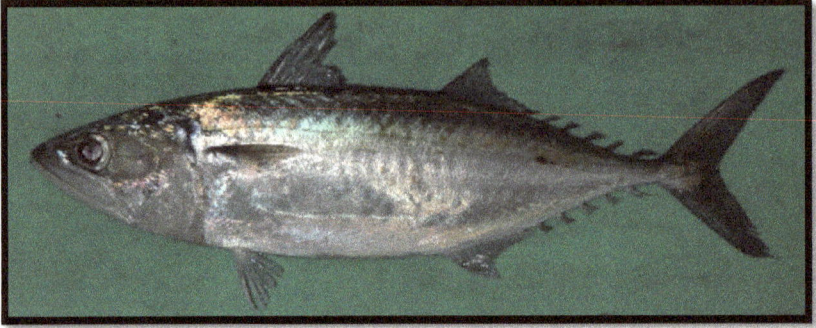

Nutritional Profile of Rastrelliger Kanagurta

Common Name: Indian Mackerel
Scientific Name: Rastrelliger kanagurta

1. Oil Content
- **Category**: Fatty
- **Oil Breakdown**: Contains about 15-20% total fat, primarily unsaturated fats.

2. Omega Fatty Acids
- **Omega-3**: Approximately 2.0-3.0g per 100g
  - Supports heart health and reduces inflammation.
- **Omega-6**: Approximately 1.0-2.0g per 100g
  - Important for skin health and cellular functions.
- **Omega-9**: Present in moderate amounts.

3. Cholesterol Content
- **Cholesterol**: About 70-90 mg per 100g
  - Moderate levels; suitable for most diets.

4. Sodium Content
- **Sodium**: Approximately 50-100 mg per 100g
  - Moderate sodium content; mindful consumption is recommended.

5. Mercury Contamination
- **Mercury Levels**: Generally low
  - Safe for regular consumption, though care should be taken in polluted waters.

6. Nutritional Information (Per 100g)
- **Calories**: ~150-200 kcal
- **Protein**: ~20-25g
  - High protein content supports muscle growth and repair.
- **Fat**: ~15-20g
  - **Saturated Fat**: ~3-5g
  - **Monounsaturated Fat**: ~5-7g
  - **Polyunsaturated Fat**: ~7-9g

7. Vitamins
- **Vitamin B12**: High (~3-5µg)
  - Essential for nerve function and red blood cell production.
- **Vitamin D**: Moderate (~200-300 IU)
  - Supports calcium absorption and bone health.
- **Vitamin B6**: Present (~0.5-1.0mg)
  - Important for amino acid metabolism.

8. Minerals
- **Selenium**: High (~30-40µg)
  - Acts as an antioxidant, supporting immune health.
- **Phosphorus**: High (~250-300mg)
  - Crucial for bone health and energy metabolism.
- **Potassium**: Moderate (~300-400mg)
  - Aids in maintaining fluid balance and regulating blood pressure.
- **Iron**: Present (~0.5-1.5mg)
  - Important for oxygen transport in the body.
- **Zinc**: Present (~0.5-1.0mg)
  - Supports immune function and wound healing.

9. Amino Acids Profile (Per 100g)	• Non-Essential Amino Acids:
• **Essential Amino Acids:**	o **Alanine**: ~1.0g
o **Histidine**: ~0.5g	o **Aspartic Acid**: ~2.5g
o **Isoleucine**: ~1.3g	o **Glutamic Acid**: ~4.0g
o **Leucine**: ~1.8g	o **Serine**: ~0.8g
o **Lysine**: ~2.5g	o **Glycine**: ~0.7g
o **Methionine**: ~0.5g	o **Proline**: ~0.5g
o **Phenylalanine**: ~0.8g	o **Tyrosine**: ~0.4g
o **Threonine**: ~0.9g	o **Cysteine**: ~0.3g
o **Tryptophan**: ~0.3g	
o **Valine**: ~1.5g	
o **Arginine**: ~1.1g	

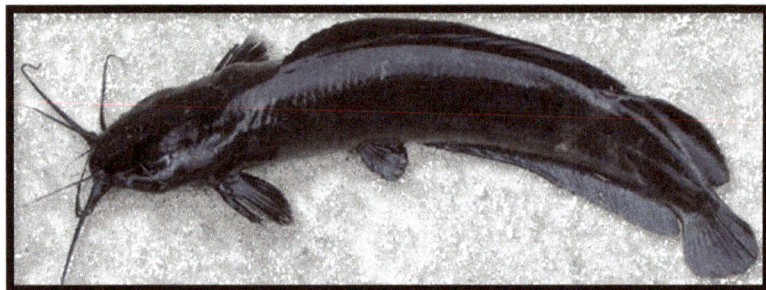

Magur

Nutritional Profile of Clarias Batrachus

Common Name: Catfish   **Scientific Name**: Clarias batrachus

1. Oil Content
- **Category**: Moderate to Fatty
- **Oil Breakdown**: Contains about 10-15% total fat, primarily unsaturated fats.

2. Omega Fatty Acids
- **Omega-3**: Approximately 0.5-1.0g per 100g
  o Supports heart health and reduces inflammation.
- **Omega-6**: Approximately 2.0-3.0g per 100g
  o Important for skin health and cellular functions.
- **Omega-9**: Present in moderate amounts.

3. Cholesterol Content
- **Cholesterol**: About 60-80 mg per 100g
  o Moderate levels; suitable for most diets.

4. Sodium Content
- **Sodium**: Approximately 50-70 mg per 100g
  o Moderate sodium content; mindful consumption is recommended.

5. Mercury Contamination
- **Mercury Levels**: Generally low
  o Safe for regular consumption, though care should be taken in polluted waters.

6. Nutritional Information (Per 100g)
- **Calories**: ~120-150 kcal

- **Protein**: ~15-20g
  - High protein content supports muscle growth and repair.
- **Fat**: ~10-15g
  - **Saturated Fat**: ~2-3g
  - **Monounsaturated Fat**: ~4-6g
  - **Polyunsaturated Fat**: ~4-6g

7. Vitamins

- **Vitamin B12**: Moderate (~2-4µg)
  - Essential for nerve function and red blood cell production.
- **Vitamin D**: Moderate (~50-100 IU)
  - Supports calcium absorption and bone health.
- **Vitamin B6**: Present (~0.5-0.8mg)
  - Important for amino acid metabolism.

8. Minerals

- **Selenium**: Moderate (~15-25µg)
  - Acts as an antioxidant, supporting immune health.
- **Phosphorus**: High (~200-250mg)
  - Crucial for bone health and energy metabolism.
- **Potassium**: Moderate (~300-350mg)
  - Aids in maintaining fluid balance and regulating blood pressure.
- **Iron**: Present (~0.5-1.0mg)
  - Important for oxygen transport in the body.
- **Zinc**: Present (~0.4-0.6mg)
  - Supports immune function and wound healing.

9. Amino Acids Profile (Per 100g)	Non-Essential Amino Acids:
Essential Amino Acids:	Alanine: ~0.9g
○ **Histidine**: ~0.5g	**Aspartic Acid**: ~2.0g
○ **Isoleucine**: ~1.2g	**Glutamic Acid**: ~3.8g
○ **Leucine**: ~1.6g	**Serine**: ~0.7g
○ **Lysine**: ~1.9g	**Glycine**: ~0.5g
○ **Methionine**: ~0.4g	**Proline**: ~0.4g
○ **Phenylalanine**: ~0.7g	**Tyrosine**: ~0.3g
○ **Threonine**: ~0.8g	**Cysteine**: ~0.2g
○ **Tryptophan**: ~0.3g	
○ **Valine**: ~1.3g	
○ **Arginine**: ~1	

   ○ .0g

Meni

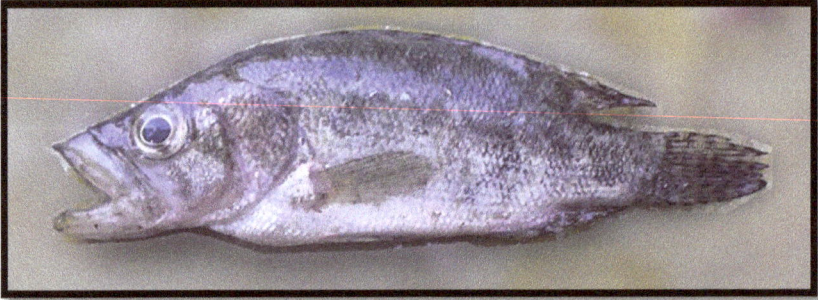

Nutritional Profile of Nandus Nandus

Common Name: Indian Nandus   **Scientific Name**: Nandus nandus

1. Oil Content
- **Category**: Moderate
- **Oil Breakdown**: Contains about 5-10% total fat, primarily unsaturated fats.

2. Omega Fatty Acids
- **Omega-3**: Approximately 0.5-1.0g per 100g
  - Supports heart health and reduces inflammation.
- **Omega-6**: Approximately 1.0-1.5g per 100g
  - Important for skin health and cellular functions.
- **Omega-9**: Present in small amounts.

3. Cholesterol Content
- **Cholesterol**: About 40-60 mg per 100g
  - Moderate levels; suitable for most diets.

4. Sodium Content
- **Sodium**: Approximately 40-70 mg per 100g
  - Moderate sodium content; mindful consumption is recommended.

5. Mercury Contamination
- **Mercury Levels**: Generally low
  - Safe for regular consumption, though care should be taken in polluted waters.

6. Nutritional Information (Per 100g)
- **Calories**: ~100-150 kcal

- **Protein**: ~15-20g
  - High protein content supports muscle growth and repair.
- **Fat**: ~5-10g
  - **Saturated Fat**: ~1-2g
  - **Monounsaturated Fat**: ~2-3g
  - **Polyunsaturated Fat**: ~2-5g

7. Vitamins

- **Vitamin B12**: Moderate (~2-4µg)
  - Essential for nerve function and red blood cell production.
- **Vitamin D**: Present (~100-200 IU)
  - Supports calcium absorption and bone health.
- **Vitamin B6**: Moderate (~0.5-0.7mg)
  - Important for amino acid metabolism.

8. Minerals

- **Selenium**: Moderate (~10-20µg)
  - Acts as an antioxidant, supporting immune health.
- **Phosphorus**: High (~150-200mg)
  - Crucial for bone health and energy metabolism.
- **Potassium**: Moderate (~250-300mg)
  - Aids in maintaining fluid balance and regulating blood pressure.
- **Iron**: Present (~0.4-1.0mg)
  - Important for oxygen transport in the body.
- **Zinc**: Present (~0.3-0.5mg)
  - Supports immune function and wound healing.

9. Amino Acids Profile (Per 100g)	
• **Essential Amino Acids**:	• **Non-Essential Amino Acids**:
○ **Histidine**: ~0.4g	○ **Alanine**: ~0.8g
○ **Isoleucine**: ~1.0g	○ **Aspartic Acid**: ~2.0g
○ **Leucine**: ~1.4g	○ **Glutamic Acid**: ~3.5g
○ **Lysine**: ~2.0g	○ **Serine**: ~0.6g
○ **Methionine**: ~0.3g	○ **Glycine**: ~0.5g
○ **Phenylalanine**: ~0.6g	○ **Proline**: ~0.4g
○ **Threonine**: ~0.7g	○ **Tyrosine**: ~0.3g
○ **Tryptophan**: ~0.3g	○ **Cysteine**: ~0.2g
○ **Valine**: ~1.2g	
○ **Arginine**: ~1.0g	

Mocca

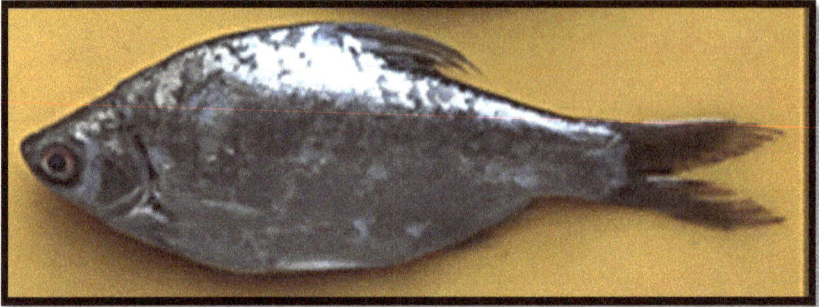

Nutritional Profile of Osteobrama Cotio

Common Name: Indian Carp   **Scientific Name**: Osteobrama cotio

1. Oil Content
- **Category**: Lean to Moderate
- **Oil Breakdown**: Contains about 3-7% total fat, primarily unsaturated fats.

2. Omega Fatty Acids
- **Omega-3**: Approximately 0.3-0.5g per 100g
  - Supports heart health and reduces inflammation.
- **Omega-6**: Approximately 0.5-1.0g per 100g
  - Important for skin health and cellular functions.
- **Omega-9**: Present in small amounts.

3. Cholesterol Content
- **Cholesterol**: About 30-50 mg per 100g
  - Low to moderate levels; suitable for most diets.

4. Sodium Content
- **Sodium**: Approximately 40-60 mg per 100g
  - Moderate sodium content; mindful consumption is recommended.

5. Mercury Contamination
- **Mercury Levels**: Generally low
  - Safe for regular consumption, though care should be taken in polluted waters.

6. Nutritional Information (Per 100g)
- **Calories**: ~90-120 kcal

- **Protein**: ~15-18g
  - High protein content supports muscle growth and repair.
- **Fat**: ~3-7g
  - **Saturated Fat**: ~0.5-1g
  - **Monounsaturated Fat**: ~1-2g
  - **Polyunsaturated Fat**: ~1-3g

7. Vitamins
- **Vitamin B12**: Moderate (~2-3μg)
  - Essential for nerve function and red blood cell production.
- **Vitamin D**: Present (~50-100 IU)
  - Supports calcium absorption and bone health.
- **Vitamin B6**: Present (~0.3-0.5mg)
  - Important for amino acid metabolism.

8. Minerals
- **Selenium**: Moderate (~10-15μg)
  - Acts as an antioxidant, supporting immune health.
- **Phosphorus**: High (~150-200mg)
  - Crucial for bone health and energy metabolism.
- **Potassium**: Moderate (~250-300mg)
  - Aids in maintaining fluid balance and regulating blood pressure.
- **Iron**: Present (~0.5-1.0mg)
  - Important for oxygen transport in the body.
- **Zinc**: Present (~0.3-0.6mg)
  - Supports immune function and wound healing.

9. Amino Acids Profile (Per 100g)	
Essential Amino Acids:	• **Non-Essential Amino Acids:**
○ **Histidine**: ~0.4g	○ **Alanine**: ~0.8g
○ **Isoleucine**: ~1.0g	○ **Aspartic Acid**: ~1.8g
○ **Leucine**: ~1.3g	○ **Glutamic Acid**: ~3.2g
○ **Lysine**: ~2.0g	○ **Serine**: ~0.5g
○ **Methionine**: ~0.3g	○ **Glycine**: ~0.4g
○ **Phenylalanine**: ~0.5g	○ **Proline**: ~0.3g
○ **Threonine**: ~0.7g	○ **Tyrosine**: ~0.3g
○ **Tryptophan**: ~0.3g	○ **Cysteine**: ~0.2g
○ **Valine**: ~1.0g	
○ **Arginine**: ~0.9g	

Mola

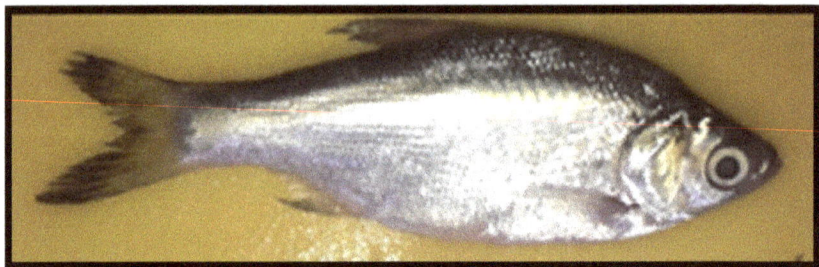

Nutritional Profile of Amblypharyngodon Mola

Common Name: Mola Fish   **Scientific Name**: Amblypharyngodon mola

1. Oil Content
- **Category**: Lean
- **Oil Breakdown**: Contains about 2-5% total fat, primarily unsaturated fats.

2. Omega Fatty Acids
- **Omega-3**: Approximately 0.2-0.4g per 100g
  - Supports heart health and reduces inflammation.
- **Omega-6**: Approximately 0.3-0.5g per 100g
  - Important for skin health and cellular functions.
- **Omega-9**: Present in small amounts.

3. Cholesterol Content
- **Cholesterol**: About 30-40 mg per 100g
  - Low levels; suitable for most diets.

4. Sodium Content
- **Sodium**: Approximately 40-60 mg per 100g
  - Moderate sodium content; mindful consumption is recommended.

5. Mercury Contamination
- **Mercury Levels**: Generally low
  - Safe for regular consumption, though care should be taken in polluted waters.

6. Nutritional Information (Per 100g)
- **Calories**: ~70-100 kcal

- **Protein**: ~15-20g
  - High protein content supports muscle growth and repair.
- **Fat**: ~2-5g
  - **Saturated Fat**: ~0.5-1g
  - **Monounsaturated Fat**: ~1-2g
  - **Polyunsaturated Fat**: ~0.5-2g

7. Vitamins

- **Vitamin B12**: Moderate (~1-2µg)
  - Essential for nerve function and red blood cell production.
- **Vitamin D**: Present (~30-50 IU)
  - Supports calcium absorption and bone health.
- **Vitamin B6**: Present (~0.2-0.4mg)
  - Important for amino acid metabolism.

8. Minerals

- **Selenium**: Moderate (~10-15µg)
  - Acts as an antioxidant, supporting immune health.
- **Phosphorus**: Moderate (~100-150mg)
  - Crucial for bone health and energy metabolism.
- **Potassium**: Moderate (~200-250mg)
  - Aids in maintaining fluid balance and regulating blood pressure.
- **Iron**: Present (~0.4-0.6mg)
  - Important for oxygen transport in the body.
- **Zinc**: Present (~0.2-0.4mg)
  - Supports immune function and wound healing.

9. Amino Acids Profile (Per 100g)	Non-Essential Amino Acids:
• **Essential Amino Acids:**	○ **Alanine**: ~0.7g
○ **Histidine**: ~0.3g	○ **Aspartic Acid**: ~1.5g
○ **Isoleucine**: ~0.9g	○ **Glutamic Acid**: ~2.5g
○ **Leucine**: ~1.2g	○ **Serine**: ~0.5g
○ **Lysine**: ~1.8g	○ **Glycine**: ~0.4g
○ **Methionine**: ~0.3g	○ **Proline**: ~0.3g
○ **Phenylalanine**: ~0.5g	○ **Tyrosine**: ~0.3g
○ **Threonine**: ~0.6g	○ **Cysteine**: ~0.2g
○ **Tryptophan**: ~0.2g	
○ **Valine**: ~1.0g	
○ **Arginine**: ~0.8g	

Mrigel

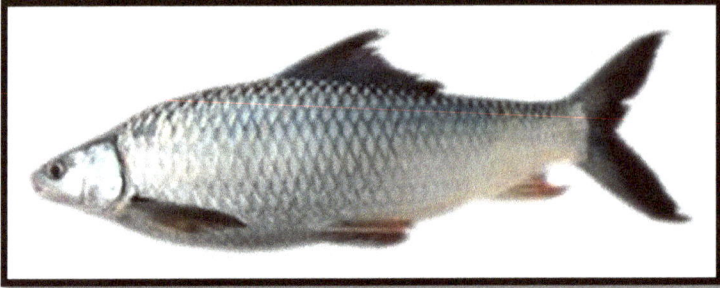

Nutritional Profile of Cirrhinus Mrigala

Common Name: Mrigal Carp   **Scientific Name**: Cirrhinus mrigala

1. Oil Content
- **Category**: Moderate
- **Oil Breakdown**: Contains about 4-8% total fat, primarily unsaturated fats.

2. Omega Fatty Acids
- **Omega-3**: Approximately 0.5-1.0g per 100g
    o   Supports heart health and reduces inflammation.
- **Omega-6**: Approximately 1.0-1.5g per 100g
    o   Important for skin health and cellular functions.
- **Omega-9**: Present in small amounts.

3. Cholesterol Content
- **Cholesterol**: About 40-60 mg per 100g
    o   Moderate levels; suitable for most diets.

4. Sodium Content
- **Sodium**: Approximately 50-70 mg per 100g
    o   Moderate sodium content; mindful consumption is recommended.

5. Mercury Contamination
- **Mercury Levels**: Generally low
    o   Safe for regular consumption, though care should be taken in polluted waters.

6. Nutritional Information (Per 100g)
- **Calories**: ~120-150 kcal
- **Protein**: ~18-22g
    o   High protein content supports muscle growth and repair.
- **Fat**: ~4-8g
    o   **Saturated Fat**: ~1-2g
    o   **Monounsaturated Fat**: ~1-3g

○   **Polyunsaturated Fat**: ~1-3g

7. Vitamins

- **Vitamin B12**: Moderate (~2-4µg)
  - ○   Essential for nerve function and red blood cell production.
- **Vitamin D**: Present (~50-100 IU)
  - ○   Supports calcium absorption and bone health.
- **Vitamin B6**: Present (~0.5-0.7mg)
  - ○   Important for amino acid metabolism.

8. Minerals

- **Selenium**: Moderate (~15-20µg)
  - ○   Acts as an antioxidant, supporting immune health.
- **Phosphorus**: High (~200-250mg)
  - ○   Crucial for bone health and energy metabolism.
- **Potassium**: Moderate (~300-350mg)
  - ○   Aids in maintaining fluid balance and regulating blood pressure.
- **Iron**: Present (~0.5-1.0mg)
  - ○   Important for oxygen transport in the body.
- **Zinc**: Present (~0.4-0.6mg)
  - ○   Supports immune function and wound healing.

9. Amino Acids Profile (Per 100g)	• Non-Essential Amino Acids:
• **Essential Amino Acids:** ○ **Histidine**: ~0.4g ○ **Isoleucine**: ~1.0g ○ **Leucine**: ~1.5g ○ **Lysine**: ~2.5g ○ **Methionine**: ~0.3g ○ **Phenylalanine**: ~0.6g ○ **Threonine**: ~0.8g ○ **Tryptophan**: ~0.3g ○ **Valine**: ~1.2g ○ **Arginine**: ~1.0g	• **Alanine**: ~0.9g • **Aspartic Acid**: ~2.0g • **Glutamic Acid**: ~3.5g • **Serine**: ~0.6g • **Glycine**: ~0.5g • **Proline**: ~0.4g • **Tyrosine**: ~0.3g • **Cysteine**: ~0.2g

Nola

Other names: Baby Mirka, Baby Mrigal   scientific name? Cirrhinus Mrigala

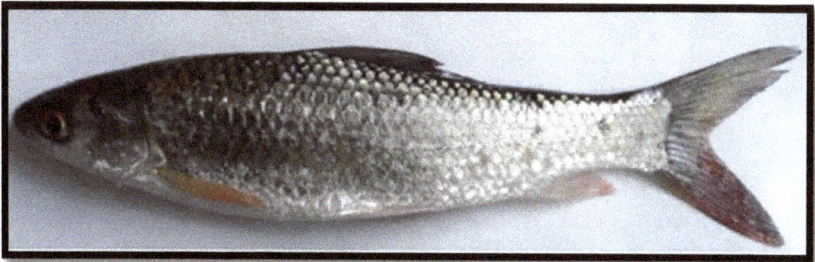

Mussel

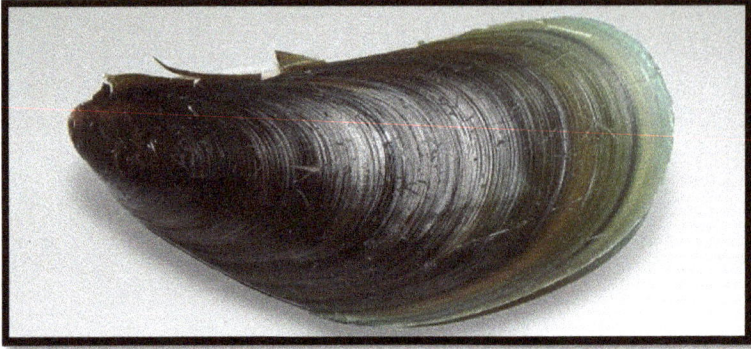

Nutritional Profile of Perna Viridis

Common Name: Green Mussel
Scientific Name: Perna viridis

1. Oil Content
- **Category**: Low
- **Oil Breakdown**: Contains about 1-2% total fat, primarily unsaturated fats.

2. Omega Fatty Acids
- **Omega-3**: Approximately 0.5-1.0g per 100g
  - Supports heart health and reduces inflammation.
- **Omega-6**: Approximately 0.1-0.3g per 100g
  - Important for skin health and cellular functions.
- **Omega-9**: Present in small amounts.

3. Cholesterol Content
- **Cholesterol**: About 40-50 mg per 100g
  - Low levels; suitable for most diets.

4. Sodium Content
- **Sodium**: Approximately 50-70 mg per 100g
  - Moderate sodium content; mindful consumption is recommended.

5. Mercury Contamination
- **Mercury Levels**: Generally low
  - Safe for regular consumption, though care should be taken in polluted waters.

6. Nutritional Information (Per 100g)
- **Calories**: ~70-90 kcal
- **Protein**: ~15-20g
  - High protein content supports muscle growth and repair.
- **Fat**: ~1-2g
  - **Saturated Fat**: ~0.2g
  - **Monounsaturated Fat**: ~0.4g
  - **Polyunsaturated Fat**: ~0.5g

7. Vitamins
- **Vitamin B12**: High (~5-8µg)
  - Essential for nerve function and red blood cell production.
- **Vitamin D**: Present (~50-100 IU)
  - Supports calcium absorption and bone health.
- **Vitamin B6**: Present (~0.2-0.5mg)
  - Important for amino acid metabolism.

8. Minerals
- **Selenium**: Moderate (~20-30µg)
  - Acts as an antioxidant, supporting immune health.
- **Phosphorus**: High (~150-200mg)
  - Crucial for bone health and energy metabolism.
- **Potassium**: Moderate (~300-350mg)
  - Aids in maintaining fluid balance and regulating blood pressure.
- **Iron**: Present (~2-3mg)
  - Important for oxygen transport in the body.
- **Zinc**: Present (~1.0-2.0mg)
  - Supports immune function and wound healing.

9. Amino Acids Profile (Per 100g)	• Non-Essential Amino Acids:
• **Essential Amino Acids**:	○ **Alanine**: ~1.0g
○ **Histidine**: ~0.6g	○ **Aspartic Acid**: ~2.2g
○ **Isoleucine**: ~1.0g	○ **Glutamic Acid**: ~3.5g
○ **Leucine**: ~1.5g	○ **Serine**: ~0.7g
○ **Lysine**: ~2.2g	○ **Glycine**: ~0.6g
○ **Methionine**: ~0.4g	○ **Proline**: ~0.5g
○ **Phenylalanine**: ~0.5g	○ **Tyrosine**: ~0.4g
○ **Threonine**: ~0.8g	○ **Cysteine**: ~0.2g
○ **Tryptophan**: ~0.2g	
○ **Valine**: ~1.1g	
○ **Arginine**: ~1.0g	

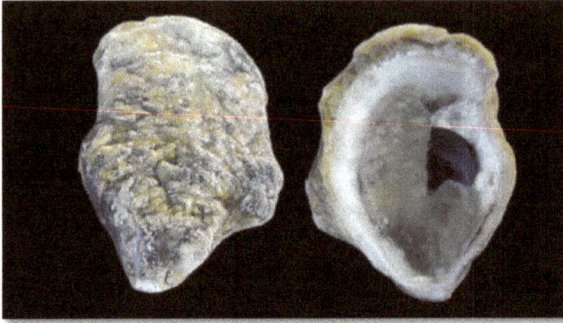

Oyster

Nutritional Profile of Crassostrea Madrasensis

Common Name: Indian Oyster   **Scientific   Name**:   Crassostrea madrasensis

1. Oil Content
- **Category**: Low
- **Oil Breakdown**: Contains about 2-4% total fat, primarily unsaturated fats.

2. Omega Fatty Acids
- **Omega-3**: Approximately 0.4-1.0g per 100g
  - o   Supports heart health and reduces inflammation.
- **Omega-6**: Approximately 0.2-0.5g per 100g
  - o   Important for skin health and cellular functions.
- **Omega-9**: Present in small amounts.

3. Cholesterol Content
- **Cholesterol**: About 40-50 mg per 100g
  - o   Low levels; suitable for most diets.

4. Sodium Content
- **Sodium**: Approximately 50-70 mg per 100g
  - o   Moderate sodium content; mindful consumption is recommended.

5. Mercury Contamination
- **Mercury Levels**: Generally low
  - o   Safe for regular consumption, though care should be taken in polluted waters.

6. Nutritional Information (Per 100g)
- Calories: ~70-90 kcal
- Protein: ~9-14g
  - High protein content supports muscle growth and repair.
- Fat: ~2-4g
  - **Saturated Fat**: ~0.5g
  - **Monounsaturated Fat**: ~0.8g
  - **Polyunsaturated Fat**: ~0.7g

7. Vitamins
- **Vitamin B12**: High (~5-8µg)
  - Essential for nerve function and red blood cell production.
- **Vitamin D**: Present (~50-100 IU)
  - Supports calcium absorption and bone health.
- **Vitamin B6**: Present (~0.2-0.5mg)
  - Important for amino acid metabolism.

8. Minerals
- **Selenium**: Moderate (~20-30µg)
  - Acts as an antioxidant, supporting immune health.
- **Phosphorus**: High (~150-200mg)
  - Crucial for bone health and energy metabolism.
- **Potassium**: Moderate (~200-300mg)
  - Aids in maintaining fluid balance and regulating blood pressure.
- **Iron**: Present (~3-5mg)
  - Important for oxygen transport in the body.
- **Zinc**: High (~2-5mg)
  - Supports immune function and wound healing.

9. Amino Acids Profile (Per 100g)		• Non-Essential Amino Acids:	
• Essential Amino Acids:			
	o Histidine: ~0.5g	o	Alanine: ~0.8g
	o Isoleucine: ~0.9g	o	Aspartic Acid: ~1.6g
	o Leucine: ~1.2g	o	Glutamic Acid: ~2.8g
	o Lysine: ~1.8g	o	Serine: ~0.5g
	o Methionine: ~0.3g	o	Glycine: ~0.5g
	o Phenylalanine: ~0.5g	o	Proline: ~0.4g
	o Threonine: ~0.6g	o	Tyrosine: ~0.3g
	o Tryptophan: ~0.2g	o	Cysteine: ~0.2g
	o Valine: ~1.0g		
	o Arginine: ~1.1g		

Pabda

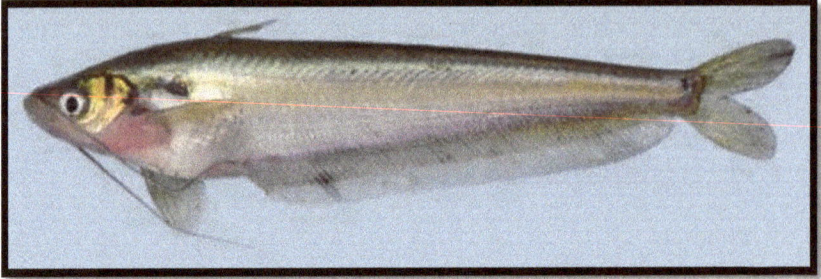

Nutritional Profile of Ompok Pabda

Common Name: Pabda Catfish   **Scientific Name**: Ompok pabda

1. Oil Content
- **Category**: Moderate
- **Oil Breakdown**: Contains about 5-10% total fat, primarily unsaturated fats.

2. Omega Fatty Acids
- **Omega-3**: Approximately 0.4-1.2g per 100g
  - o Supports heart health and reduces inflammation.
- **Omega-6**: Approximately 1.0-1.5g per 100g
  - o Important for skin health and cellular functions.
- **Omega-9**: Present in small amounts.

3. Cholesterol Content
- **Cholesterol**: About 60-70 mg per 100g
  - o Moderate levels; suitable for most diets.

4. Sodium Content
- **Sodium**: Approximately 50-80 mg per 100g
  - o Moderate sodium content; mindful consumption is recommended.

5. Mercury Contamination
- **Mercury Levels**: Generally low
  - o Safe for regular consumption, though care should be taken in polluted waters.

6. Nutritional Information (Per 100g)
- **Calories**: ~120-150 kcal

- **Protein**: ~18-22g
  - High protein content supports muscle growth and repair.
- **Fat**: ~5-10g
  - **Saturated Fat**: ~1-2g
  - **Monounsaturated Fat**: ~1-3g
  - **Polyunsaturated Fat**: ~2-5g

7. Vitamins

- **Vitamin B12**: High (~3-6µg)
  - Essential for nerve function and red blood cell production.
- **Vitamin D**: Present (~50-100 IU)
  - Supports calcium absorption and bone health.
- **Vitamin B6**: Present (~0.5-0.7mg)
  - Important for amino acid metabolism.

8. Minerals

- **Selenium**: Moderate (~15-25µg)
  - Acts as an antioxidant, supporting immune health.
- **Phosphorus**: High (~200-250mg)
  - Crucial for bone health and energy metabolism.
- **Potassium**: Moderate (~300-350mg)
  - Aids in maintaining fluid balance and regulating blood pressure.
- **Iron**: Present (~1-2mg)
  - Important for oxygen transport in the body.
- **Zinc**: Present (~0.6-1.2mg)
  - Supports immune function and wound healing.

9. Amino Acids Profile (Per 100g)	Non-Essential Amino Acids:
Essential Amino Acids:	
○ **Histidine**: ~0.5g	○ **Alanine**: ~1.0g
○ **Isoleucine**: ~1.1g	○ **Aspartic Acid**: ~2.0g
○ **Leucine**: ~1.5g	○ **Glutamic Acid**: ~3.0g
○ **Lysine**: ~2.5g	○ **Serine**: ~0.7g
○ **Methionine**: ~0.4g	○ **Glycine**: ~0.5g
○ **Phenylalanine**: ~0.6g	○ **Proline**: ~0.4g
○ **Threonine**: ~0.8g	○ **Tyrosine**: ~0.3g
○ **Tryptophan**: ~0.3g	○ **Cysteine**: ~0.2g
○ **Valine**: ~1.2g	
○ **Arginine**: ~1.0g	

Pangush

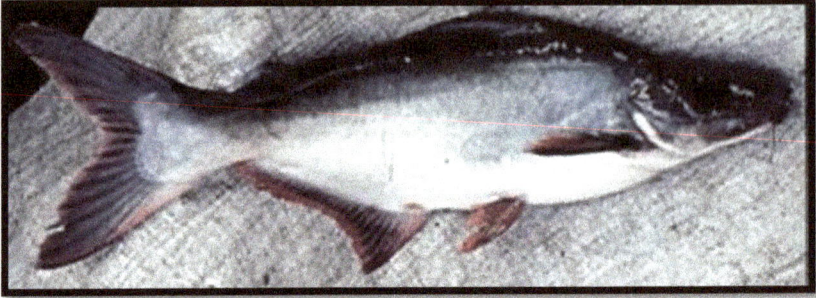

Nutritional Profile of Pangasius Pangasius

Common Name: Pangasius Catfish
Scientific Name: Pangasius pangasius

1. Oil Content
- **Category**: Moderate
- **Oil Breakdown**: Contains about 4-8% total fat, primarily unsaturated fats.

2. Omega Fatty Acids
- **Omega-3**: Approximately 0.5-1.0g per 100g
  - Supports heart health and reduces inflammation.
- **Omega-6**: Approximately 2.5-3.0g per 100g
  - Important for skin health and cellular functions.
- **Omega-9**: Present in small amounts.

3. Cholesterol Content
- **Cholesterol**: About 50-70 mg per 100g
  - Moderate levels; suitable for most diets.

4. Sodium Content
- **Sodium**: Approximately 60-80 mg per 100g
  - Moderate sodium content; mindful consumption is recommended.

5. Mercury Contamination
- **Mercury Levels**: Generally low
  - Safe for regular consumption, although care should be taken in polluted waters.

6. Nutritional Information (Per 100g)
- **Calories**: ~90-120 kcal
- **Protein**: ~15-20g
  - High protein content supports muscle growth and repair.
- **Fat**: ~4-8g
  - **Saturated Fat**: ~1-2g
  - **Monounsaturated Fat**: ~1-3g
  - **Polyunsaturated Fat**: ~2-5g

7. Vitamins
- **Vitamin B12**: Moderate (~2-4µg)
  - Essential for nerve function and red blood cell production.
- **Vitamin D**: Present (~50-80 IU)
  - Supports calcium absorption and bone health.
- **Vitamin B6**: Present (~0.3-0.5mg)
  - Important for amino acid metabolism.

8. Minerals
- **Selenium**: Moderate (~20-30µg)
  - Acts as an antioxidant, supporting immune health.
- **Phosphorus**: High (~200-250mg)
  - Crucial for bone health and energy metabolism.
- **Potassium**: Moderate (~300-350mg)
  - Aids in maintaining fluid balance and regulating blood pressure.
- **Iron**: Present (~0.5-1.0mg)
  - Important for oxygen transport in the body.
- **Zinc**: Present (~0.8-1.2mg)
  - Supports immune function and wound healing.

9. Amino Acids Profile (Per 100g)	Non-Essential Amino Acids:
Essential Amino Acids: ○ **Histidine**: ~0.5g ○ **Isoleucine**: ~1.0g ○ **Leucine**: ~1.4g ○ **Lysine**: ~1.9g ○ **Methionine**: ~0.3g ○ **Phenylalanine**: ~0.6g ○ **Threonine**: ~0.7g ○ **Tryptophan**: ~0.3g ○ **Valine**: ~1.1g ○ **Arginine**: ~1.2g	○ **Alanine**: ~0.8g ○ **Aspartic Acid**: ~1.6g ○ **Glutamic Acid**: ~3.0g ○ **Serine**: ~0.6g ○ **Glycine**: ~0.4g ○ **Proline**: ~0.5g ○ **Tyrosine**: ~0.3g ○ **Cysteine**: ~0.2g

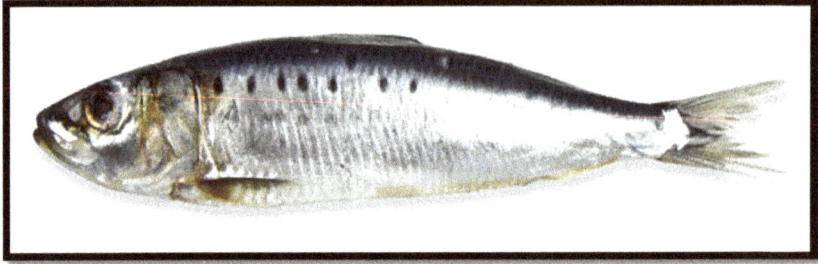

Pilchard

Nutritional Profile of Pilchard

Common Name: Pilchard
Scientific Name: Sardinus pilchardus (commonly referred to as European Pilchard)

1. Oil Content
- **Category**: Fatty
- **Oil Breakdown**: Contains about 10-20% total fat, primarily unsaturated fats.

2. Omega Fatty Acids
- **Omega-3**: Approximately 1.5-2.5g per 100g
  - Supports heart health and reduces inflammation.
- **Omega-6**: Approximately 0.5-1.0g per 100g
  - Important for skin health and cellular functions.
- **Omega-9**: Present in moderate amounts.

3. Cholesterol Content
- **Cholesterol**: About 50-60 mg per 100g
  - Moderate levels; suitable for most diets.

4. Sodium Content
- **Sodium**: Approximately 60-80 mg per 100g (varies with processing)
  - Moderate sodium content; mindful consumption is recommended.

5. Mercury Contamination
- **Mercury Levels**: Generally low
  - Safe for regular consumption, though care should be taken in polluted waters.

6. Nutritional Information (Per 100g)
- **Calories**: ~150-200 kcal
- **Protein**: ~20-25g
  - High protein content supports muscle growth and repair.
- **Fat**: ~10-20g
  - **Saturated Fat**: ~1-3g
  - **Monounsaturated Fat**: ~2-4g
  - **Polyunsaturated Fat**: ~4-10g

7. Vitamins
- **Vitamin B12**: High (~8-10µg)
  - Essential for nerve function and red blood cell production.
- **Vitamin D**: Present (~500-600 IU)
  - Supports calcium absorption and bone health.
- **Vitamin B6**: Present (~0.5-1.0mg)
  - Important for amino acid metabolism.

8. Minerals
- **Selenium**: Moderate (~30-40µg)
  - Acts as an antioxidant, supporting immune health.
- **Phosphorus**: High (~200-250mg)
  - Crucial for bone health and energy metabolism.
- **Potassium**: Moderate (~300-400mg)
  - Aids in maintaining fluid balance and regulating blood pressure.
- **Iron**: Present (~1-2mg)
  - Important for oxygen transport in the body.
- **Zinc**: Present (~1.0-1.5mg)
  - Supports immune function and wound healing.

9. Amino Acids Profile (Per 100g)	Non-Essential Amino Acids:
Essential Amino Acids:	
Histidine: ~0.5g	Alanine: ~1.0g
Isoleucine: ~1.2g	Aspartic Acid: ~2.0g
Leucine: ~1.8g	Glutamic Acid: ~4.0g
Lysine: ~2.7g	Serine: ~0.8g
Methionine: ~0.4g	Glycine: ~0.6g
Phenylalanine: ~0.7g	Proline: ~0.5g
Threonine: ~0.9g	Tyrosine: ~0.4g
Tryptophan: ~0.3g	Cysteine: ~0.3g
Valine: ~1.2g	
Arginine: ~1.0g	

Pomfret Black

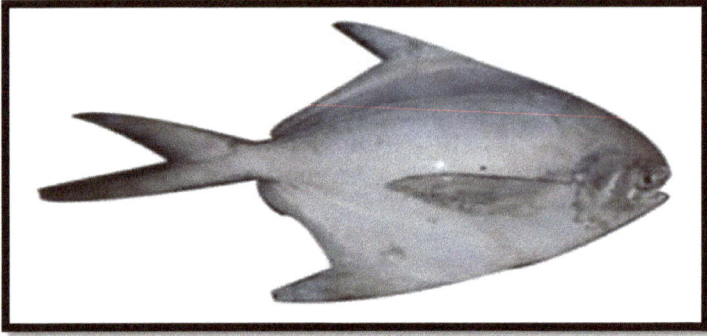

Nutritional Profile of Parastromateus Niger

Common Name: Black Pomfret
Scientific Name: Parastromateus niger

1. Oil Content
- **Category**: Moderate to High
- **Oil Breakdown**: Contains about 10-15% total fat, primarily unsaturated fats.

2. Omega Fatty Acids
- **Omega-3**: Approximately 1.0-1.5g per 100g
  - Supports heart health and reduces inflammation.
- **Omega-6**: Approximately 1.5-2.5g per 100g
  - Important for skin health and cellular functions.
- **Omega-9**: Present in moderate amounts.

3. Cholesterol Content
- **Cholesterol**: About 60-80 mg per 100g
  - Moderate levels; suitable for most diets.

4. Sodium Content
- **Sodium**: Approximately 50-70 mg per 100g
  - Moderate sodium content; mindful consumption is recommended.

5. Mercury Contamination
- **Mercury Levels**: Generally low
  - Safe for regular consumption, though care should be taken in polluted waters.

6. Nutritional Information (Per 100g)
- **Calories**: ~120-150 kcal
- **Protein**: ~20-25g
  - High protein content supports muscle growth and repair.
- **Fat**: ~10-15g
  - **Saturated Fat**: ~2-3g
  - **Monounsaturated Fat**: ~3-5g
  - **Polyunsaturated Fat**: ~3-5g

7. Vitamins
- **Vitamin B12**: High (~4-6µg)
  - Essential for nerve function and red blood cell production.
- **Vitamin D**: Present (~100-150 IU)
  - Supports calcium absorption and bone health.
- **Vitamin B6**: Present (~0.5-0.8mg)
  - Important for amino acid metabolism.

8. Minerals
- **Selenium**: Moderate (~25-35µg)
  - Acts as an antioxidant, supporting immune health.
- **Phosphorus**: High (~200-250mg)
  - Crucial for bone health and energy metabolism.
- **Potassium**: Moderate (~300-400mg)
  - Aids in maintaining fluid balance and regulating blood pressure.
- **Iron**: Present (~1-2mg)
  - Important for oxygen transport in the body.
- **Zinc**: Present (~0.8-1.5mg)
  - Supports immune function and wound healing.

9. Amino Acids Profile (Per 100g)	• Non-Essential Amino Acids:
• **Essential Amino Acids**:	o **Alanine**: ~0.9g
o **Histidine**: ~0.5g	o **Aspartic Acid**: ~1.8g
o **Isoleucine**: ~1.1g	o **Glutamic Acid**: ~3.5g
o **Leucine**: ~1.8g	o **Serine**: ~0.7g
o **Lysine**: ~2.3g	o **Glycine**: ~0.5g
o **Methionine**: ~0.4g	o **Proline**: ~0.6g
o **Phenylalanine**: ~0.6g	o **Tyrosine**: ~0.4g
o **Threonine**: ~0.9g	o **Cysteine**: ~0.2g
o **Tryptophan**: ~0.3g	
o **Valine**: ~1.2g	
o **Arginine**: ~1.1g	

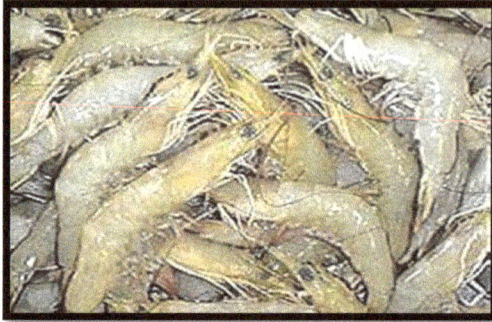

Prawn Indian

Nutritional Profile of Fenneropenaeus Indicus

Common Name: Indian White Shrimp
Scientific Name: Fenneropenaeus indicus

1. Oil Content
- **Category**: Low to Moderate
- **Oil Breakdown**: Contains about 1-3% total fat, primarily unsaturated fats.

2. Omega Fatty Acids
- **Omega-3**: Approximately 0.3-0.6g per 100g
  - o Supports heart health and reduces inflammation.
- **Omega-6**: Approximately 0.5-1.0g per 100g
  - o Important for skin health and cellular functions.
- **Omega-9**: Present in small amounts.

3. Cholesterol Content
- **Cholesterol**: About 150-200 mg per 100g
  - o Moderate levels; should be consumed in moderation.

4. Sodium Content
- **Sodium**: Approximately 70-90 mg per 100g
  - o Moderate sodium content; mindful consumption is recommended.

5. Mercury Contamination
- **Mercury Levels**: Generally low
  - o Safe for regular consumption, though care should be taken in polluted waters.

6. Nutritional Information (Per 100g)
- **Calories**: ~85-100 kcal
- **Protein**: ~18-22g
  - High protein content supports muscle growth and repair.
- **Fat**: ~1-3g
  - **Saturated Fat**: <1g
  - **Monounsaturated Fat**: ~0.2-0.5g
  - **Polyunsaturated Fat**: ~0.5-1g

7. Vitamins
- **Vitamin B12**: Moderate (~2-4µg)
  - Essential for nerve function and red blood cell production.
- **Vitamin E**: Present (~0.5-1mg)
  - Acts as an antioxidant, protecting cells from damage.
- **Vitamin B6**: Present (~0.3-0.6mg)
  - Important for amino acid metabolism.

8. Minerals
- **Selenium**: Moderate (~20-30µg)
  - Acts as an antioxidant, supporting immune health.
- **Phosphorus**: High (~200-250mg)
  - Crucial for bone health and energy metabolism.
- **Potassium**: Moderate (~250-300mg)
  - Aids in maintaining fluid balance and regulating blood pressure.
- **Iron**: Present (~1-2mg)
  - Important for oxygen transport in the body.
- **Zinc**: Present (~1.0-1.5mg)
  - Supports immune function and wound healing.

9. Amino Acids Profile (Per 100g)	
Essential Amino Acids:	• **Non-Essential Amino Acids:**
○ **Histidine**: ~0.5g	○ **Alanine**: ~0.8g
○ **Isoleucine**: ~1.0g	○ **Aspartic Acid**: ~1.7g
○ **Leucine**: ~1.6g	○ **Glutamic Acid**: ~3.4g
○ **Lysine**: ~2.5g	○ **Serine**: ~0.7g
○ **Methionine**: ~0.5g	○ **Glycine**: ~0.6g
○ **Phenylalanine**: ~0.6g	○ **Proline**: ~0.5g
○ **Threonine**: ~0.8g	○ **Tyrosine**: ~0.4g
○ **Tryptophan**: ~0.3g	○ **Cysteine**: ~0.2g
○ **Valine**: ~1.1g	
○ **Arginine**: ~1.0g	

Prawns, Tiger Prawn Indian

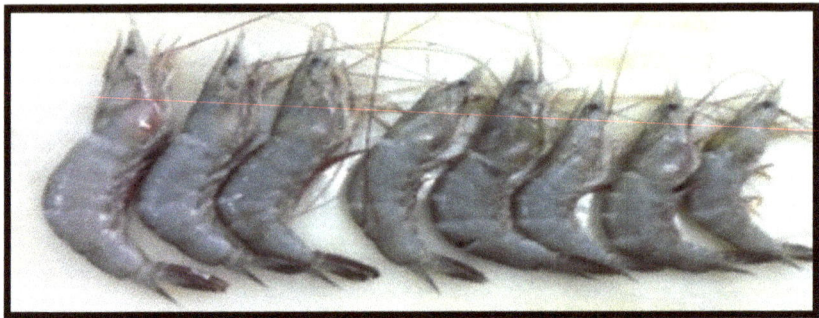

Nutritional Profile of Penaeus Monodon

Common Name: Black Tiger Shrimp
Scientific Name: Penaeus monodon

1. Oil Content
- **Category**: Low to Moderate
- **Oil Breakdown**: Contains about 1-3% total fat, primarily unsaturated fats.

2. Omega Fatty Acids
- **Omega-3**: Approximately 0.5-1.0g per 100g
  o Supports heart health and reduces inflammation.
- **Omega-6**: Approximately 0.5-1.0g per 100g
  o Important for skin health and cellular functions.
- **Omega-9**: Present in small amounts.

3. Cholesterol Content
- **Cholesterol**: About 150-200 mg per 100g
  o Moderate levels; should be consumed in moderation.

4. Sodium Content
- **Sodium**: Approximately 60-80 mg per 100g
  o Moderate sodium content; mindful consumption is recommended.

5. Mercury Contamination
- **Mercury Levels**: Generally low
  o Safe for regular consumption, though care should be taken in polluted waters.

6. Nutritional Information (Per 100g)
- Calories: ~80-100 kcal
- Protein: ~18-24g
  - High protein content supports muscle growth and repair.
- Fat: ~1-3g
  - **Saturated Fat**: <1g
  - **Monounsaturated Fat**: ~0.2-0.5g
  - **Polyunsaturated Fat**: ~0.5-1g

7. Vitamins
- **Vitamin B12**: Moderate (~2-4µg)
  - Essential for nerve function and red blood cell production.
- **Vitamin E**: Present (~0.5-1mg)
  - Acts as an antioxidant, protecting cells from damage.
- **Vitamin B6**: Present (~0.3-0.6mg)
  - Important for amino acid metabolism.

8. Minerals
- **Selenium**: Moderate (~20-30µg)
  - Acts as an antioxidant, supporting immune health.
- **Phosphorus**: High (~200-250mg)
  - Crucial for bone health and energy metabolism.
- **Potassium**: Moderate (~250-300mg)
  - Aids in maintaining fluid balance and regulating blood pressure.
- **Iron**: Present (~1-2mg)
  - Important for oxygen transport in the body.
- **Zinc**: Present (~1.0-1.5mg)
  - Supports immune function and wound healing.

9. Amino Acids Profile (Per 100g)	Non-Essential Amino Acids:
• Essential Amino Acids:	
○ **Histidine**: ~0.5g	○ **Alanine**: ~0.9g
○ **Isoleucine**: ~1.0g	○ **Aspartic Acid**: ~1.7g
○ **Leucine**: ~1.5g	○ **Glutamic Acid**: ~3.4g
○ **Lysine**: ~2.5g	○ **Serine**: ~0.7g
○ **Methionine**: ~0.5g	○ **Glycine**: ~0.6g
○ **Phenylalanine**: ~0.6g	○ **Proline**: ~0.5g
○ **Threonine**: ~0.8g	○ **Tyrosine**: ~0.4g
○ **Tryptophan**: ~0.3g	○ **Cysteine**: ~0.3g
○ **Valine**: ~1.1g	
○ **Arginine**: ~1.2g	

Puti (Ticto)

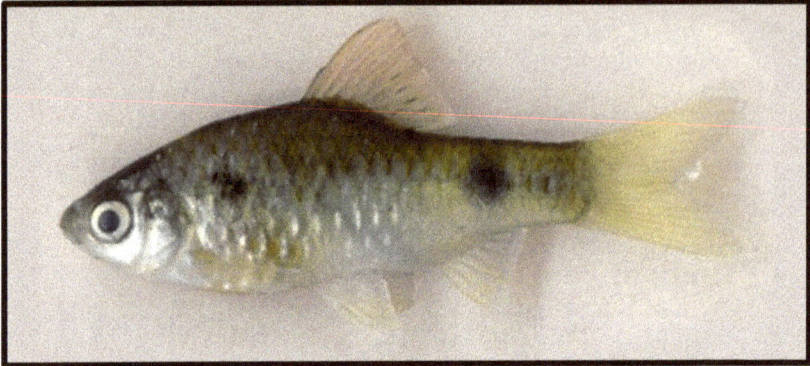

Nutritional Profile of Puntius ticto

Common Name: Ticto Barb   **Scientific Name**: Puntius ticto

1. Oil Content
- **Category**: Medium-fat
- **Oil Breakdown**: Approximately 3-5% total fat, primarily unsaturated fats.

2. Omega Fatty Acids
- **Omega-3**: About 0.3-0.5g per 100g
  o Supports heart health and reduces inflammation.
- **Omega-6**: Approximately 0.2-0.4g per 100g
  o Important for skin health and cellular functions.
- **Omega-9**: Present in moderate amounts.

3. Cholesterol Content
- **Cholesterol**: About 50-70 mg per 100g
  o Moderate levels; generally acceptable for most diets.

4. Sodium Content
- **Sodium**: Approximately 30-50 mg per 100g
  o Low sodium content; beneficial for blood pressure management.

5. Mercury Contamination
- **Mercury Levels**: Low
  o Generally safe for consumption with minimal risk of mercury contamination.

6. Nutritional Information (Per 100g)
- **Calories**: ~90-110 kcal
- **Protein**: ~17-19g
  - High protein content supports muscle growth and repair.
- **Fat**: ~3-5g
  - **Saturated Fat**: ~0.8-1.0g
  - **Monounsaturated Fat**: ~1.0-1.2g
  - **Polyunsaturated Fat**: ~1.2-1.5g

7. Vitamins
- **Vitamin B12**: Moderate (~1.5-3μg)
  - Essential for nerve function and red blood cell production.
- **Vitamin D**: Present (~5-10 IU)
  - Important for bone health and calcium absorption.
- **Vitamin B6**: Present (~0.3-0.5mg)
  - Important for amino acid metabolism.

8. Minerals
- **Selenium**: Moderate (~15-25μg)
  - Acts as an antioxidant, supporting immune health.
- **Phosphorus**: Moderate (~130-180mg)
  - Crucial for bone health and energy metabolism.
- **Potassium**: Moderate (~180-230mg)
  - Aids in maintaining fluid balance and regulating blood pressure.
- **Iron**: Present (~0.6-0.9mg)
  - Important for oxygen transport in the body.

9. Amino Acids Profile (Per 100g) • **Essential Amino Acids:**	• **Non-Essential Amino Acids:**
○ **Histidine**: ~0.3g	○ **Alanine**: ~0.5g
○ **Isoleucine**: ~0.8g	○ **Aspartic Acid**: ~1.1g
○ **Leucine**: ~1.3g	
○ **Lysine**: ~1.5g	○ **Glutamic Acid**: ~1.8g
○ **Methionine**: ~0.3g	
○ **Phenylalanine**: ~0.6g	○ **Serine**: ~0.4g
○ **Threonine**: ~0.7g	○ **Glycine**: ~0.4g
○ **Tryptophan**: ~0.1g	○ **Proline**: ~0.3g
○ **Valine**: ~0.8g	○ **Tyrosine**: ~0.2g
○ **Arginine**: ~0.8g	○ **Cysteine**: ~0.2g

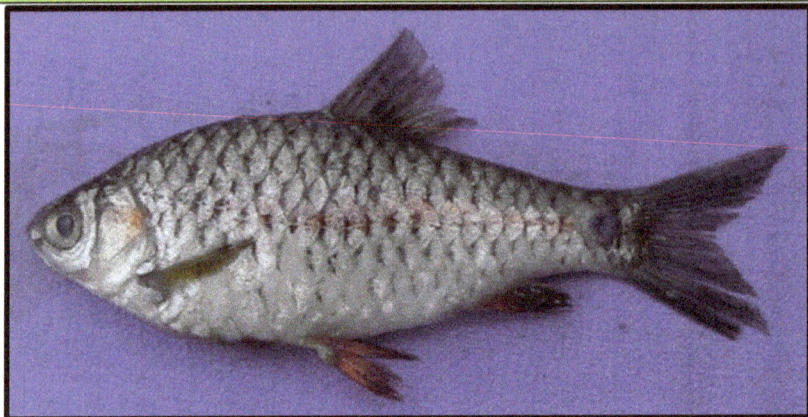

Puti

Nutritional Profile of Puntius Sophore

Common Name: Sophore Fish
Scientific Name: Puntius sophore

1. Oil Content
- **Category**: Lean
- **Oil Breakdown**: Approximately 1-2% total fat, primarily unsaturated fats.

2. Omega Fatty Acids
- **Omega-3**: About 0.2-0.4g per 100g
  - Supports heart health and has anti-inflammatory properties.
- **Omega-6**: Approximately 0.3-0.5g per 100g
  - Important for skin health and cellular functions.
- **Omega-9**: Present in small amounts.

3. Cholesterol Content
- **Cholesterol**: About 50-70 mg per 100g
  - Low to moderate levels; suitable for most diets.

4. Sodium Content
- **Sodium**: Approximately 40-60 mg per 100g
  - Low sodium content; beneficial for hypertension management.

5. Mercury Contamination
- **Mercury Levels**: Generally low
  - Safe for regular consumption.

6. Nutritional Information (Per 100g)
- **Calories**: ~70-80 kcal
- **Protein**: ~15-20g
  - High protein content supports muscle growth and repair.
- **Fat**: ~1-2g
  - **Saturated Fat**: <0.5g
  - **Monounsaturated Fat**: ~0.1-0.2g
  - **Polyunsaturated Fat**: ~0.5g

7. Vitamins
- **Vitamin B12**: Moderate (~1-2µg)
  - Essential for nerve function and red blood cell production.
- **Vitamin D**: Present in small amounts
  - Important for bone health.
- **Vitamin B6**: Present (~0.2-0.4mg)
  - Important for amino acid metabolism.

8. Minerals
- **Selenium**: Moderate (~15-25µg)
  - Acts as an antioxidant, supporting immune health.
- **Phosphorus**: Moderate (~150-200mg)
  - Crucial for bone health and energy metabolism.
- **Potassium**: Moderate (~200-250mg)
  - Aids in maintaining fluid balance and regulating blood pressure.
- **Iron**: Present (~0.5-1mg)
  - Important for oxygen transport in the body.

9. Amino Acids Profile (Per 100g)	
Essential Amino Acids:	• **Non-Essential Amino Acids:**
○ **Histidine**: ~0.4g	○ **Alanine**: ~0.6g
○ **Isoleucine**: ~0.8g	○ **Aspartic Acid**: ~1.3g
○ **Leucine**: ~1.2g	○ **Glutamic Acid**: ~2.5g
○ **Lysine**: ~1.5g	○ **Serine**: ~0.5g
○ **Methionine**: ~0.3g	○ **Glycine**: ~0.4g
○ **Phenylalanine**: ~0.5g	○ **Proline**: ~0.3g
○ **Threonine**: ~0.6g	○ **Tyrosine**: ~0.3g
○ **Tryptophan**: ~0.2g	○ **Cysteine**: ~0.1g
○ **Valine**: ~0.9g	
○ **Arginine**: ~0.7g	

Puti, Shor

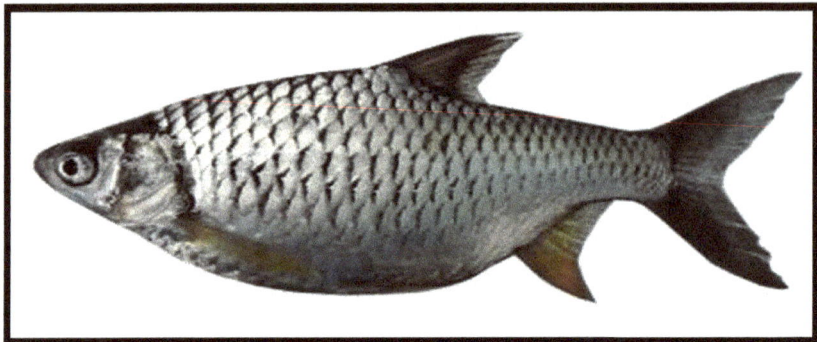

Nutritional Profile of Tor Putitora

Common Name: Golden Mahseer
Scientific Name: Tor putitora

1. Oil Content
- **Category**: Moderate
- **Oil Breakdown**: Approximately 5-10% total fat, predominantly unsaturated fats.

2. Omega Fatty Acids
- **Omega-3**: About 0.8-1.2g per 100g
  - Supports heart health and reduces inflammation.
- **Omega-6**: Approximately 1-2g per 100g
  - Important for skin health and cellular functions.
- **Omega-9**: Present in moderate amounts.

3. Cholesterol Content
- **Cholesterol**: About 70-90 mg per 100g
  - Moderate levels; generally acceptable for most diets.

4. Sodium Content
- **Sodium**: Approximately 40-60 mg per 100g
  - Low sodium content; beneficial for blood pressure management.

5. Mercury Contamination
- **Mercury Levels**: Generally low
  - Safe for regular consumption.

6. Nutritional Information (Per 100g)
- Calories: ~120-150 kcal
- Protein: ~20-25g
  - High protein content supports muscle growth and repair.
- Fat: ~5-10g
  - **Saturated Fat**: ~1-2g
  - **Monounsaturated Fat**: ~1-3g
  - **Polyunsaturated Fat**: ~1-2g

7. Vitamins
- **Vitamin B12**: Moderate (~2-3µg)
  - Essential for nerve function and red blood cell production.
- **Vitamin D**: Present in small amounts
  - Important for bone health and calcium absorption.
- **Vitamin B6**: Present (~0.5-0.8mg)
  - Important for amino acid metabolism.

8. Minerals
- **Selenium**: Moderate (~25-35µg)
  - Acts as an antioxidant, supporting immune health.
- **Phosphorus**: High (~250-300mg)
  - Crucial for bone health and energy metabolism.
- **Potassium**: Moderate (~250-300mg)
  - Aids in maintaining fluid balance and regulating blood pressure.
- **Iron**: Present (~1-2mg)
  - Important for oxygen transport in the body.
- **Zinc**: Present (~1.5-2mg)
  - Supports immune function and wound healing.

9. Amino Acids Profile (Per 100g)	Non-Essential Amino Acids:
Essential Amino Acids:	
○ **Histidine**: ~0.6g	○ **Alanine**: ~0.7g
○ **Isoleucine**: ~1.1g	○ **Aspartic Acid**: ~1.5g
○ **Leucine**: ~1.6g	○ **Glutamic Acid**: ~3.0g
○ **Lysine**: ~2.4g	○ **Serine**: ~0.6g
○ **Methionine**: ~0.4g	○ **Glycine**: ~0.5g
○ **Phenylalanine**: ~0.7g	○ **Proline**: ~0.4g
○ **Threonine**: ~0.9g	○ **Tyrosine**: ~0.4g
○ **Tryptophan**: ~0.3g	○ **Cysteine**: ~0.2g
○ **Valine**: ~1.2g	
○ **Arginine**: ~1.0g	

Rani

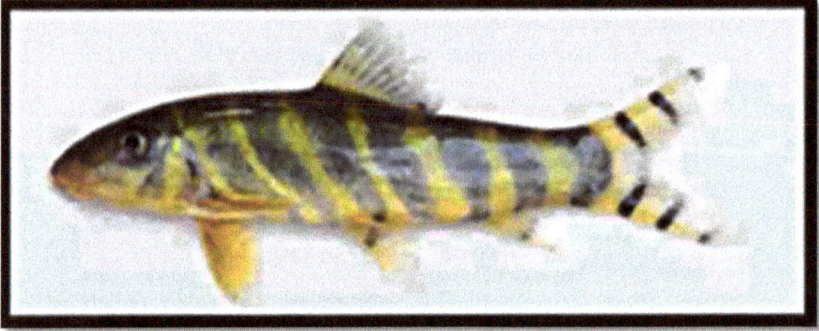

Nutritional Profile of Botia Dario

Common Name: Dario Loach
Scientific Name: Botia Dario

1. Oil Content
- **Category**: Lean
- **Oil Breakdown**: Approximately 1-2% total fat, primarily unsaturated fats.

2. Omega Fatty Acids
- **Omega-3**: About 0.3-0.5g per 100g
  - Supports heart health and has anti-inflammatory properties.
- **Omega-6**: Approximately 0.4-0.6g per 100g
  - Important for skin health and cellular functions.
- **Omega-9**: Present in small amounts.

3. Cholesterol Content
- **Cholesterol**: About 50-60 mg per 100g
  - Low levels; suitable for most diets.

4. Sodium Content
- **Sodium**: Approximately 30-50 mg per 100g
  - Low sodium content; beneficial for hypertension management.

5. Mercury Contamination
- **Mercury Levels**: Generally low
  - Safe for regular consumption.

6. Nutritional Information (Per 100g)
- **Calories**: ~80-90 kcal

- **Protein**: ~15-18g
  - High protein content supports muscle growth and repair.
- **Fat**: ~1-2g
  - **Saturated Fat**: <0.5g
  - **Monounsaturated Fat**: ~0.2g
  - **Polyunsaturated Fat**: ~0.4g

7. Vitamins

- **Vitamin B12**: Moderate (~1-2μg)
  - Essential for nerve function and red blood cell production.
- **Vitamin D**: Present in small amounts
  - Important for bone health and calcium absorption.
- **Vitamin B6**: Present (~0.2-0.4mg)
  - Important for amino acid metabolism.

8. Minerals

- **Selenium**: Moderate (~15-25μg)
  - Acts as an antioxidant, supporting immune health.
- **Phosphorus**: Moderate (~150-200mg)
  - Crucial for bone health and energy metabolism.
- **Potassium**: Moderate (~200-250mg)
  - Aids in maintaining fluid balance and regulating blood pressure.
- **Iron**: Present (~0.5-1mg)
  - Important for oxygen transport in the body.

9. Amino Acids Profile (Per 100g)	Non-Essential Amino Acids:
Essential Amino Acids:	
○ **Histidine**: ~0.5g	○ **Alanine**: ~0.6g
○ **Isoleucine**: ~0.8g	○ **Aspartic Acid**: ~1.4g
○ **Leucine**: ~1.3g	○ **Glutamic Acid**: ~2.5g
○ **Lysine**: ~1.8g	○ **Serine**: ~0.5g
○ **Methionine**: ~0.3g	○ **Glycine**: ~0.4g
○ **Phenylalanine**: ~0.6g	○ **Proline**: ~0.3g
○ **Threonine**: ~0.7g	○ **Tyrosine**: ~0.4g
○ **Tryptophan**: ~0.3g	○ **Cysteine**: ~0.2g
○ **Valine**: ~1.0g	
○ **Arginine**: ~0.8g	

Rita

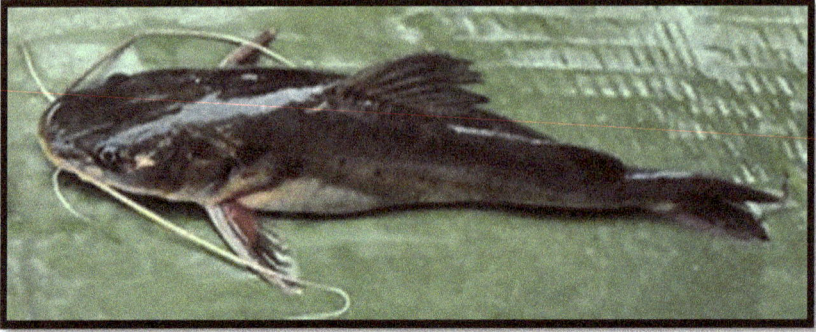

Nutritional Profile of Rita Rita

Common Name: Rita Fish   **Scientific Name**: Rita rita

1. Oil Content
- **Category**: Moderate
- **Oil Breakdown**: Approximately 5-8% total fat, primarily unsaturated fats.

2. Omega Fatty Acids
- **Omega-3**: About 0.5-1.0g per 100g
  - o Supports cardiovascular health and reduces inflammation.
- **Omega-6**: Approximately 1.0-1.5g per 100g
  - o Important for skin health and cellular functions.
- **Omega-9**: Present in moderate amounts.

3. Cholesterol Content
- **Cholesterol**: About 60-80 mg per 100g
  - o Moderate levels; generally acceptable for most diets.

4. Sodium Content
- **Sodium**: Approximately 50-70 mg per 100g
  - o Low sodium content; beneficial for blood pressure management.

5. Mercury Contamination
- **Mercury Levels**: Generally low
  - o Safe for regular consumption.

6. Nutritional Information (Per 100g)
- **Calories**: ~120-140 kcal

- **Protein**: ~20-22g
  - High protein content supports muscle growth and repair.
- **Fat**: ~5-8g
  - **Saturated Fat**: ~1-2g
  - **Monounsaturated Fat**: ~1-3g
  - **Polyunsaturated Fat**: ~2-3g

7. Vitamins

- **Vitamin B12**: Moderate (~2-3µg)
  - Essential for nerve function and red blood cell production.
- **Vitamin D**: Present in small amounts
  - Important for bone health and calcium absorption.
- **Vitamin B6**: Present (~0.5-0.7mg)
  - Important for amino acid metabolism.

8. Minerals

- **Selenium**: Moderate (~20-30µg)
  - Acts as an antioxidant, supporting immune health.
- **Phosphorus**: High (~200-250mg)
  - Crucial for bone health and energy metabolism.
- **Potassium**: Moderate (~250-300mg)
  - Aids in maintaining fluid balance and regulating blood pressure.
- **Iron**: Present (~1-2mg)
  - Important for oxygen transport in the body.

9. Amino Acids Profile (Per 100g) • **Essential Amino Acids:**	• **Non-Essential Amino Acids:**
o **Histidine**: ~0.5g	o **Alanine**: ~0.7g
o **Isoleucine**: ~1.0g	o **Aspartic Acid**: ~1.5g
o **Leucine**: ~1.6g	o **Glutamic Acid**: ~3.0g
o **Lysine**: ~2.1g	o **Serine**: ~0.6g
o **Methionine**: ~0.4g	o **Glycine**: ~0.5g
o **Phenylalanine**: ~0.7g	o **Proline**: ~0.4g
o **Threonine**: ~0.9g	o **Tyrosine**: ~0.4g
o **Tryptophan**: ~0.3g	**Cysteine**: ~0.2g
o **Valine**: ~1.1g	
o **Arginine**: ~0.9g	

Rohu

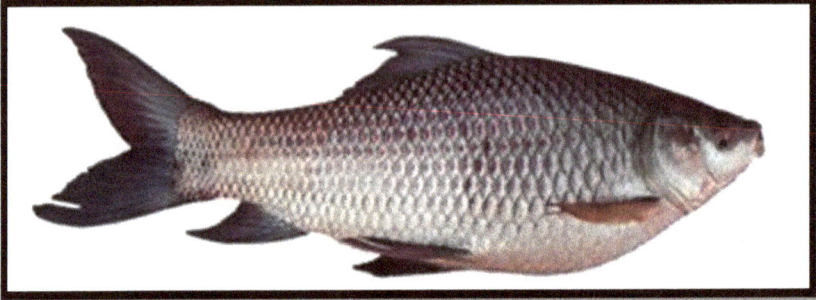

Nutritional Profile of Labeo Rohita

Common Name: Rohu   **Scientific Name**: Labeo rohita

1. Oil Content
- **Category**: Moderate
- **Oil Breakdown**: Approximately 5-10% total fat, primarily unsaturated fats.

2. Omega Fatty Acids
- **Omega-3**: About 0.6-1.0g per 100g
  - o   Supports cardiovascular health and reduces inflammation.
- **Omega-6**: Approximately 1.5-2.5g per 100g
  - o   Important for skin health and cellular functions.
- **Omega-9**: Present in moderate amounts.

3. Cholesterol Content
- **Cholesterol**: About 70-90 mg per 100g
  - o   Moderate levels; generally acceptable for most diets.

4. Sodium Content
- **Sodium**: Approximately 50-70 mg per 100g
  - o   Low sodium content; beneficial for blood pressure management.

5. Mercury Contamination
- **Mercury Levels**: Generally low
  - o   Safe for regular consumption.

6. Nutritional Information (Per 100g)
- **Calories**: ~120-150 kcal

- **Protein**: ~20-25g
  - High protein content supports muscle growth and repair.
- **Fat**: ~5-10g
  - **Saturated Fat**: ~1-2g
  - **Monounsaturated Fat**: ~1-3g
  - **Polyunsaturated Fat**: ~2-4g

7. Vitamins
- **Vitamin B12**: Moderate (~2-3μg)
  - Essential for nerve function and red blood cell production.
- **Vitamin D**: Present in small amounts
  - Important for bone health and calcium absorption.
- **Vitamin B6**: Present (~0.4-0.6mg)
  - Important for amino acid metabolism.

8. Minerals
- **Selenium**: Moderate (~20-30μg)
  - Acts as an antioxidant, supporting immune health.
- **Phosphorus**: High (~200-250mg)
  - Crucial for bone health and energy metabolism.
- **Potassium**: Moderate (~250-300mg)
  - Aids in maintaining fluid balance and regulating blood pressure.
- **Iron**: Present (~1-2mg)
  - Important for oxygen transport in the body.

9. Amino Acids Profile (Per 100g)	
Essential Amino Acids:	• **Non-Essential Amino Acids:**
○ **Histidine**: ~0.5g	○ **Alanine**: ~0.8g
○ **Isoleucine**: ~1.1g	○ **Aspartic Acid**: ~1.5g
○ **Leucine**: ~1.7g	○ **Glutamic Acid**: ~3.2g
○ **Lysine**: ~2.4g	○ **Serine**: ~0.7g
○ **Methionine**: ~0.5g	○ **Glycine**: ~0.6g
○ **Phenylalanine**: ~0.8g	○ **Proline**: ~0.5g
○ **Threonine**: ~1.0g	○ **Tyrosine**: ~0.5g
○ **Tryptophan**: ~0.3g	○ **Cysteine**: ~0.3g
○ **Valine**: ~1.2g	
○ **Arginine**: ~1.0g	

Salmon, Atlantic

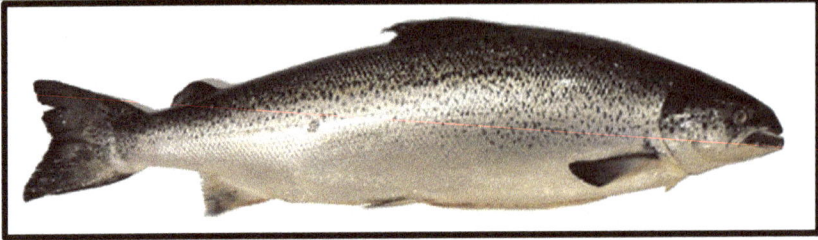

Nutritional Profile of Salmo Salar

Common Name: Atlantic Salmon   **Scientific Name**: Salmo salar

1. Oil Content
- **Category**: Fatty
- **Oil Breakdown**: Approximately 13-20% total fat, primarily unsaturated fats.

2. Omega Fatty Acids
- **Omega-3**: About 2.0-3.0g per 100g
  - Supports cardiovascular health and reduces inflammation.
- **Omega-6**: Approximately 0.5-1.0g per 100g
  - Important for skin health and cellular functions.
- **Omega-9**: Present in significant amounts.

3. Cholesterol Content
- **Cholesterol**: About 60-70 mg per 100g
  - Moderate levels; generally acceptable for most diets.

4. Sodium Content
- **Sodium**: Approximately 50-60 mg per 100g
  - Low sodium content; beneficial for blood pressure management.

5. Mercury Contamination
- **Mercury Levels**: Generally low
  - Safe for regular consumption.

6. Nutritional Information (Per 100g)
- **Calories**: ~206 kcal
- **Protein**: ~20-25g
  - High protein content supports muscle growth and repair.

- **Fat**: ~13-20g
  - **Saturated Fat**: ~3-4g
  - **Monounsaturated Fat**: ~5-7g
  - **Polyunsaturated Fat**: ~4-6g

7. Vitamins
- **Vitamin B12**: High (~3-4μg)
  - Essential for nerve function and red blood cell production.
- **Vitamin D**: High (~10-15μg)
  - Important for bone health and calcium absorption.
- **Vitamin B6**: Present (~0.8-1.0mg)
  - Important for amino acid metabolism.

8. Minerals
- **Selenium**: High (~30-50μg)
  - Acts as an antioxidant, supporting immune health.
- **Phosphorus**: Moderate (~200-250mg)
  - Crucial for bone health and energy metabolism.
- **Potassium**: Moderate (~300-350mg)
  - Aids in maintaining fluid balance and regulating blood pressure.
- **Iron**: Present (~0.5-1.0mg)
  - Important for oxygen transport in the body.

9. Amino Acids Profile (Per 100g)	•Non-Essential Amino Acids:
Essential Amino Acids:	o **Alanine**: ~0.9g
o **Histidine**: ~0.5g	o **Aspartic Acid**: ~1.5g
o **Isoleucine**: ~1.1g	o **Glutamic Acid**: ~3.5g
o **Leucine**: ~1.6g	o **Serine**: ~0.7g
o **Lysine**: ~2.3g	o **Glycine**: ~0.6g
o **Methionine**: ~0.7g	o **Proline**: ~0.4g
o **Phenylalanine**: ~1.0g	o **Tyrosine**: ~0.6g
o **Threonine**: ~1.0g	o **Cysteine**: ~0.3g
o **Tryptophan**: ~0.3g	
o **Valine**: ~1.2g	
o **Arginine**: ~1.1g	

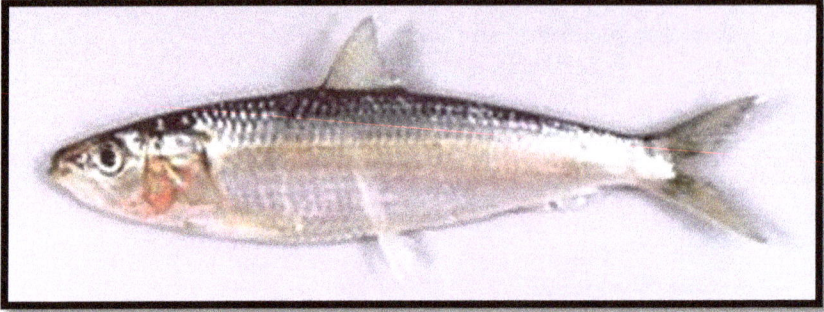
Sardine

Nutritional Profile of Sardinella Longiceps

Common Name: Longfin Sardine
Scientific Name: Sardinella longiceps

1. Oil Content
- **Category**: Fatty
- **Oil Breakdown**: Approximately 8-15% total fat, primarily unsaturated fats.

2. Omega Fatty Acids
- **Omega-3**: About 1.5-2.5g per 100g
  - Supports cardiovascular health and reduces inflammation.
- **Omega-6**: Approximately 0.5-1.0g per 100g
  - Important for skin health and cellular functions.
- **Omega-9**: Present in moderate amounts.

3. Cholesterol Content
- **Cholesterol**: About 40-60 mg per 100g
  - Moderate levels; generally acceptable for most diets.

4. Sodium Content
- **Sodium**: Approximately 60-80 mg per 100g
  - Low sodium content; beneficial for blood pressure management.

5. Mercury Contamination
- **Mercury Levels**: Generally low
  - Safe for regular consumption.

6. Nutritional Information (Per 100g)
- **Calories**: ~150-180 kcal
- **Protein**: ~20-25g
  - High protein content supports muscle growth and repair.
- **Fat**: ~8-15g
  - **Saturated Fat**: ~1-2g
  - **Monounsaturated Fat**: ~2-3g
  - **Polyunsaturated Fat**: ~5-10g

7. Vitamins
- **Vitamin B12**: High (~8-10µg)
  - Essential for nerve function and red blood cell production.
- **Vitamin D**: Moderate (~2-3µg)
  - Important for bone health and calcium absorption.
- **Vitamin B6**: Present (~0.5-0.7mg)
  - Important for amino acid metabolism.

8. Minerals
- **Selenium**: High (~30-40µg)
  - Acts as an antioxidant, supporting immune health.
- **Phosphorus**: Moderate (~200mg)
  - Crucial for bone health and energy metabolism.
- **Potassium**: Moderate (~300mg)
  - Aids in maintaining fluid balance and regulating blood pressure.
- **Iron**: Present (~1-2mg)
  - Important for oxygen transport in the body.

9. Amino Acids Profile (Per 100g)	Non-Essential Amino Acids:
Essential Amino Acids:	
Histidine: ~0.5g	**Alanine**: ~0.9g
Isoleucine: ~1.1g	**Aspartic Acid**: ~1.5g
Leucine: ~1.6g	**Glutamic Acid**: ~3.2g
Lysine: ~2.4g	**Serine**: ~0.7g
Methionine: ~0.5g	**Glycine**: ~0.6g
Phenylalanine: ~1.0g	**Proline**: ~0.5g
Threonine: ~1.0g	**Tyrosine**: ~0.6g
Tryptophan: ~0.3g	**Cysteine**: ~0.3g
Valine: ~1.2g	
Arginine: ~1.0g	

Shilong

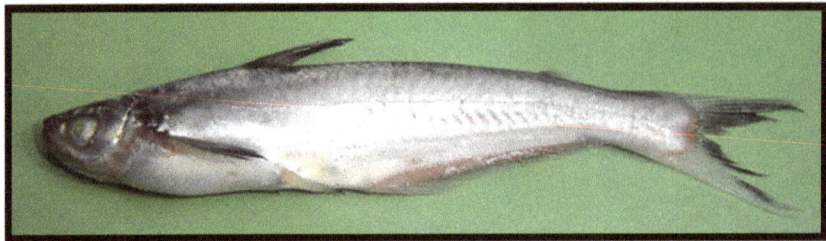

Nutritional Profile of Silonia Silondia

Common Name: Indian Schilbe   **Scientific Name**: Silonia silondia

1. Oil Content
- **Category**: Lean to Moderate
- **Oil Breakdown**: Approximately 5-10% total fat, primarily unsaturated fats.

2. Omega Fatty Acids
- **Omega-3**: About 0.5-1.0g per 100g
  - Supports cardiovascular health and reduces inflammation.
- **Omega-6**: Approximately 1.0-2.0g per 100g
  - Important for skin health and cellular functions.
- **Omega-9**: Present in smaller amounts.

3. Cholesterol Content
- **Cholesterol**: About 50-70 mg per 100g
  - Moderate levels; generally acceptable for most diets.

4. Sodium Content
- **Sodium**: Approximately 40-60 mg per 100g
  - Low sodium content; beneficial for blood pressure management.

5. Mercury Contamination
- **Mercury Levels**: Generally low
  - Safe for regular consumption.

6. Nutritional Information (Per 100g)
- **Calories**: ~130-150 kcal

- **Protein**: ~20-22g
  - High protein content supports muscle growth and repair.
- **Fat**: ~5-10g
  - **Saturated Fat**: ~1-2g
  - **Monounsaturated Fat**: ~1-3g
  - **Polyunsaturated Fat**: ~2-5g

7. Vitamins

- **Vitamin B12**: Moderate (~2-3µg)
  - Essential for nerve function and red blood cell production.
- **Vitamin D**: Present in small amounts
  - Important for bone health and calcium absorption.
- **Vitamin B6**: Present (~0.4-0.5mg)
  - Important for amino acid metabolism.

8. Minerals

- **Selenium**: Moderate (~20-30µg)
  - Acts as an antioxidant, supporting immune health.
- **Phosphorus**: Moderate (~150-200mg)
  - Crucial for bone health and energy metabolism.
- **Potassium**: Moderate (~250-300mg)
  - Aids in maintaining fluid balance and regulating blood pressure.
- **Iron**: Present (~1-1.5mg)
  - Important for oxygen transport in the body.

9. Amino Acids Profile (Per 100g)	
Essential Amino Acids: ○ **Histidine**: ~0.5g ○ **Isoleucine**: ~1.0g ○ **Leucine**: ~1.5g ○ **Lysine**: ~2.0g ○ **Methionine**: ~0.5g ○ **Phenylalanine**: ~0.8g ○ **Threonine**: ~0.9g ○ **Tryptophan**: ~0.3g ○ **Valine**: ~1.0g ○ **Arginine**: ~1.0g	• **Non-Essential Amino Acids:** ○ **Alanine**: ~0.7g ○ **Aspartic Acid**: ~1.3g ○ **Glutamic Acid**: ~2.8g ○ **Serine**: ~0.6g ○ **Glycine**: ~0.5g ○ **Proline**: ~0.4g ○ **Tyrosine**: ~0.5g ○ **Cysteine**: ~0.3g

Shing

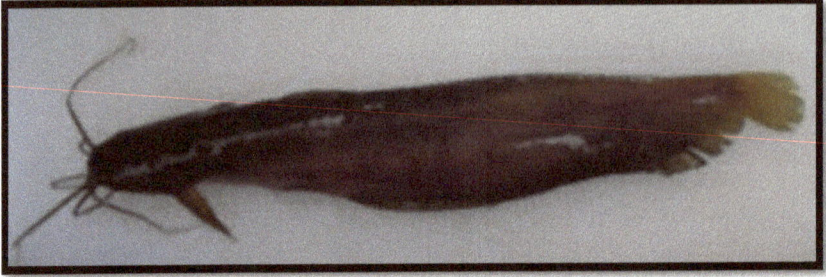

Nutritional Profile of Heteropneustes Fossilis

Common Name: Walking Catfish   **Scientific Name**: Heteropneustes fossilis

1. Oil Content
- **Category**: Lean
- **Oil Breakdown**: Approximately 2-5% total fat, primarily unsaturated fats.

2. Omega Fatty Acids
- **Omega-3**: About 0.3-0.6g per 100g
    - Supports cardiovascular health and reduces inflammation.
- **Omega-6**: Approximately 0.5-1.0g per 100g
    - Important for skin health and cellular functions.
- **Omega-9**: Present in smaller amounts.

3. Cholesterol Content
- **Cholesterol**: About 50-60 mg per 100g
    - Moderate levels; generally acceptable for most diets.

4. Sodium Content
- **Sodium**: Approximately 40-50 mg per 100g
    - Low sodium content; beneficial for blood pressure management.

5. Mercury Contamination
- **Mercury Levels**: Generally low
    - Safe for regular consumption.

6. Nutritional Information (Per 100g)
- **Calories**: ~100-120 kcal

- **Protein**: ~20-22g
  - High protein content supports muscle growth and repair.
- **Fat**: ~2-5g
  - **Saturated Fat**: ~0.5g
  - **Monounsaturated Fat**: ~0.5-1.0g
  - **Polyunsaturated Fat**: ~1-3g

7. Vitamins

- **Vitamin B12**: Moderate (~2-3µg)
  - Essential for nerve function and red blood cell production.
- **Vitamin D**: Present in small amounts
  - Important for bone health and calcium absorption.
- **Vitamin B6**: Present (~0.4-0.5mg)
  - Important for amino acid metabolism.

8. Minerals

- **Selenium**: Moderate (~20-25µg)
  - Acts as an antioxidant, supporting immune health.
- **Phosphorus**: Moderate (~150mg)
  - Crucial for bone health and energy metabolism.
- **Potassium**: Moderate (~250-300mg)
  - Aids in maintaining fluid balance and regulating blood pressure.
- **Iron**: Present (~1-1.5mg)
  - Important for oxygen transport in the body.

9. Amino Acids Profile (Per 100g)	• Non-Essential Amino Acids:
• **Essential Amino Acids:**	
○ **Histidine**: ~0.5g	○ **Alanine**: ~0.7g
○ **Isoleucine**: ~1.0g	○ **Aspartic Acid**: ~1.4g
○ **Leucine**: ~1.5g	○ **Glutamic Acid**: ~2.7g
○ **Lysine**: ~2.0g	○ **Serine**: ~0.6g
○ **Methionine**: ~0.4g	○ **Glycine**: ~0.5g
○ **Phenylalanine**: ~0.8g	○ **Proline**: ~0.4g
○ **Threonine**: ~0.9g	○ **Tyrosine**: ~0.5g
○ **Tryptophan**: ~0.3g	○ **Cysteine**: ~0.2g
○ **Valine**: ~1.1g	
○ **Arginine**: ~0.9g	

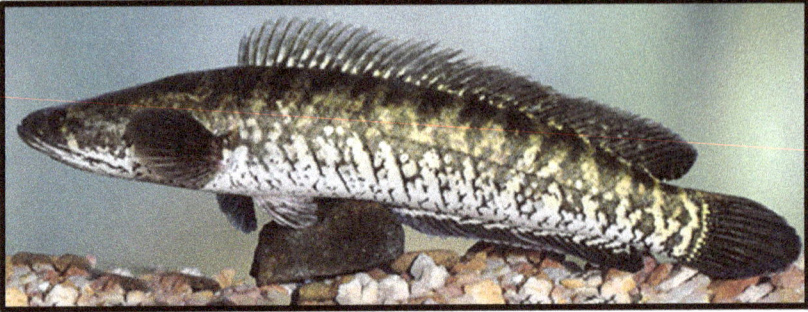

Shoil

Nutritional Profile of Channa striata

Common Name: Striped Snakehead, Snakehead Murrel
Scientific Name: Channa striata

1. Oil Content
- **Category**: Medium-fat
- **Oil Breakdown**: Approximately 4-6% total fat, primarily unsaturated fats.

2. Omega Fatty Acids
- **Omega-3**: About 0.4-0.6g per 100g
  - Supports heart health and reduces inflammation.
- **Omega-6**: Approximately 0.3-0.5g per 100g
  - Important for skin health and cellular functions.
- **Omega-9**: Present in moderate amounts.

3. Cholesterol Content
- **Cholesterol**: About 50-70 mg per 100g
  - Moderate levels; generally acceptable for most diets.

4. Sodium Content
- **Sodium**: Approximately 40-60 mg per 100g
  - Low sodium content; beneficial for blood pressure management.

5. Mercury Contamination
- **Mercury Levels**: Low
  - Generally safe for consumption with minimal risk of mercury contamination.

6. Nutritional Information (Per 100g)
- Calories: ~100-120 kcal
- Protein: ~18-20g
  - High protein content supports muscle growth and repair.
- Fat: ~4-6g
  - **Saturated Fat**: ~1.0-1.2g
  - **Monounsaturated Fat**: ~1.0-1.3g
  - **Polyunsaturated Fat**: ~1.5-1.8g

7. Vitamins
- **Vitamin B12**: Moderate (~2-4µg)
  - Essential for nerve function and red blood cell production.
- **Vitamin D**: Present (~10-20 IU)
  - Important for bone health and calcium absorption.
- **Vitamin B6**: Present (~0.4-0.6mg)
  - Important for amino acid metabolism.

8. Minerals
- **Selenium**: Moderate (~20-30µg)
  - Acts as an antioxidant, supporting immune health.
- **Phosphorus**: Moderate (~150-200mg)
  - Crucial for bone health and energy metabolism.
- **Potassium**: Moderate (~200-250mg)
  - Aids in maintaining fluid balance and regulating blood pressure.
- **Iron**: Present (~0.7-1.0mg)
  - Important for oxygen transport in the body.

9. Amino Acids Profile (Per 100g)	Non-Essential Amino Acids:
Essential Amino Acids:	•
○ **Histidine**: ~0.4g	○ **Alanine**: ~0.6g
○ **Isoleucine**: ~0.9g	○ **Aspartic Acid**: ~1.2g
○ **Leucine**: ~1.4g	○ **Glutamic Acid**: ~2.0g
○ **Lysine**: ~1.6g	○ **Serine**: ~0.5g
○ **Methionine**: ~0.4g	○ **Glycine**: ~0.5g
○ **Phenylalanine**: ~0.7g	○ **Proline**: ~0.4g
○ **Threonine**: ~0.8g	○ **Tyrosine**: ~0.3g
○ **Tryptophan**: ~0.2g	○ **Cysteine**: ~0.2g
○ **Valine**: ~0.9g	
○ **Arginine**: ~0.9g	

Shor Puti (Sarana)

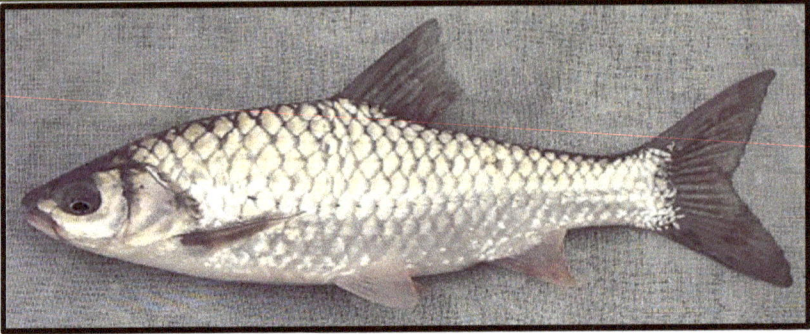

Nutritional Profile of Puntius sarana

Common Name: Olive Barb   **Scientific Name**: Puntius sarana

1. Oil Content
- **Category**: Medium-fat
- **Oil Breakdown**: Approximately 4-6% total fat, primarily unsaturated fats.

2. Omega Fatty Acids
- **Omega-3**: About 0.4-0.6g per 100g
  - Supports heart health and reduces inflammation.
- **Omega-6**: Approximately 0.3-0.5g per 100g
  - Important for skin health and cellular functions.
- **Omega-9**: Present in moderate amounts.

3. Cholesterol Content
- **Cholesterol**: About 60-80 mg per 100g
  - Moderate levels; generally acceptable for most diets.

4. Sodium Content
- **Sodium**: Approximately 40-60 mg per 100g
  - Low sodium content; beneficial for blood pressure management.

5. Mercury Contamination
- **Mercury Levels**: Low
  - Generally safe for consumption with minimal risk of mercury contamination.

6. Nutritional Information (Per 100g)

- **Calories**: ~110-130 kcal
- **Protein**: ~18-20g
  - High protein content supports muscle growth and repair.
- **Fat**: ~4-6g
  - **Saturated Fat**: ~1.0-1.2g
  - **Monounsaturated Fat**: ~1.2-1.5g
  - **Polyunsaturated Fat**: ~1.5-1.8g

7. Vitamins

- **Vitamin B12**: Moderate (~2-4µg)
  - Essential for nerve function and red blood cell production.
- **Vitamin D**: Present (~10-20 IU)
  - Important for bone health and calcium absorption.
- **Vitamin B6**: Present (~0.4-0.6mg)
  - Important for amino acid metabolism.

8. Minerals

- **Selenium**: Moderate (~20-30µg)
  - Acts as an antioxidant, supporting immune health.
- **Phosphorus**: Moderate (~150-200mg)
  - Crucial for bone health and energy metabolism.
- **Potassium**: Moderate (~200-250mg)
  - Aids in maintaining fluid balance and regulating blood pressure.
- **Iron**: Present (~0.7-1.0mg)
  - Important for oxygen transport in the body.

9. Amino Acids Profile (Per 100g)	• Non-Essential Amino
• Essential Amino Acids:	Acids:
○ Histidine: ~0.4g	○ Alanine: ~0.6g
○ Isoleucine: ~0.9g	○ Aspartic Acid: ~1.2g
○ Leucine: ~1.4g	○ Glutamic Acid: ~2.0g
○ Lysine: ~1.6g	○ Serine: ~0.5g
○ Methionine: ~0.4g	○ Glycine: ~0.5g
○ Phenylalanine: ~0.7g	○ Proline: ~0.4g
○ Threonine: ~0.8g	○ Tyrosine: ~0.3g
○ Tryptophan: ~0.2g	○ Cysteine: ~0.2g
○ Valine: ~0.9g	
○ Arginine: ~0.9g	

Silver Belly

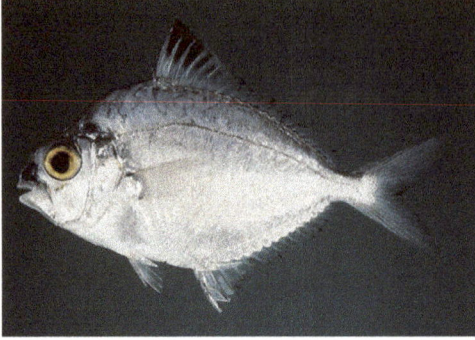

Nutritional Profile of Leiognathus splendens

Common Name: Silver Belly, Ponyfish   **Scientific   Name**:   Leiognathus
splendens

1. Oil Content
- **Category**: Medium-fat
- **Oil Breakdown**: Approximately 5-7% total fat, primarily unsaturated
  fats.

2. Omega Fatty Acids
- **Omega-3**: About 0.5-0.7g per 100g
    o   Supports heart health and reduces inflammation.
- **Omega-6**: Approximately 0.2-0.4g per 100g
    o   Important for skin health and cellular functions.
- **Omega-9**: Present in moderate amounts.

3. Cholesterol Content
- **Cholesterol**: About 60-80 mg per 100g
    o   Moderate levels; generally acceptable for most diets.

4. Sodium Content
- **Sodium**: Approximately 50-70 mg per 100g
    o   Low sodium content; beneficial for blood pressure
        management.

5. Mercury Contamination
- **Mercury Levels**: Low to moderate
    o   Generally safe for consumption but should be limited for
        pregnant women and young children.

6. Nutritional Information (Per 100g)
- **Calories**: ~110-130 kcal
- **Protein**: ~17-19g
  - High protein content supports muscle growth and repair.
- **Fat**: ~5-7g
  - **Saturated Fat**: ~1.0-1.3g
  - **Monounsaturated Fat**: ~1.5-2.0g
  - **Polyunsaturated Fat**: ~2.0-2.5g

7. Vitamins
- **Vitamin B12**: Moderate (~3-4µg)
  - Essential for nerve function and red blood cell production.
- **Vitamin D**: Present (~10-15 IU)
  - Important for bone health and calcium absorption.
- **Vitamin B6**: Present (~0.4-0.6mg)
  - Important for amino acid metabolism.

8. Minerals
- **Selenium**: Moderate (~25-35µg)
  - Acts as an antioxidant, supporting immune health.
- **Phosphorus**: Moderate (~180-220mg)
  - Crucial for bone health and energy metabolism.
- **Potassium**: Moderate (~250-300mg)
  - Aids in maintaining fluid balance and regulating blood pressure.
- **Iron**: Present (~0.7-1.1mg)
  - Important for oxygen transport in the body.

9. Amino Acids Profile (Per 100g)	• Non-Essential Amino Acids:
• **Essential Amino Acids:**	o **Alanine**: ~0.6g
o **Histidine**: ~0.4g	o **Aspartic Acid**: ~1.2g
o **Isoleucine**: ~0.9g	o **Glutamic Acid**: ~2.0g
o **Leucine**: ~1.4g	o **Serine**: ~0.5g
o **Lysine**: ~1.6g	o **Glycine**: ~0.5g
o **Methionine**: ~0.4g	o **Proline**: ~0.4g
o **Phenylalanine**: ~0.7g	o **Tyrosine**: ~0.3g
o **Threonine**: ~0.8g	o **Cysteine**: ~0.2g
o **Tryptophan**: ~0.2g	
o **Valine**: ~0.9g	
o **Arginine**: ~0.9g	

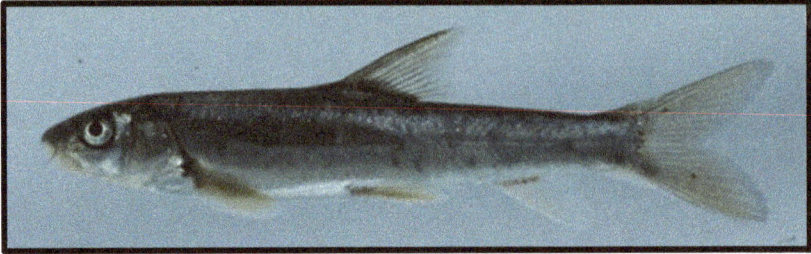

Snow Trout

Nutritional Profile of Schizothorax richardsonii

Common Name: Snow Trout, Ngaka
Scientific Name: Schizothorax richardsonii

1. Oil Content
- **Category**: Lean to medium-fat
- **Oil Breakdown**: Approximately 3-5% total fat, primarily unsaturated fats.

2. Omega Fatty Acids
- **Omega-3**: About 0.4-0.7g per 100g
  - Supports heart health and reduces inflammation.
- **Omega-6**: Approximately 0.2-0.4g per 100g
  - Important for skin health and cellular functions.
- **Omega-9**: Present in small amounts.

3. Cholesterol Content
- **Cholesterol**: About 50-70 mg per 100g
  - Moderate levels; generally acceptable for most diets.

4. Sodium Content
- **Sodium**: Approximately 40-60 mg per 100g
  - Low sodium content; beneficial for blood pressure management.

5. Mercury Contamination
- **Mercury Levels**: Low
  - Generally safe for consumption with minimal risk of mercury contamination.

6. Nutritional Information (Per 100g)
- **Calories**: ~90-110 kcal

- **Protein:** ~18-20g
  - High protein content supports muscle growth and repair.
- **Fat:** ~3-5g
  - **Saturated Fat:** ~0.8-1.0g
  - **Monounsaturated Fat:** ~1.0-1.5g
  - **Polyunsaturated Fat:** ~1.0-1.5g

7. Vitamins

- **Vitamin B12:** Moderate (~2-4μg)
  - Essential for nerve function and red blood cell production.
- **Vitamin D:** Present (~10-20 IU)
  - Important for bone health and calcium absorption.
- **Vitamin B6:** Present (~0.3-0.5mg)
  - Important for amino acid metabolism.

8. Minerals

- **Selenium:** Moderate (~20-30μg)
  - Acts as an antioxidant, supporting immune health.
- **Phosphorus:** Moderate (~150-200mg)
  - Crucial for bone health and energy metabolism.
- **Potassium:** Moderate (~200-250mg)
  - Aids in maintaining fluid balance and regulating blood pressure.
- **Iron:** Present (~0.8-1.0mg)
  - Important for oxygen transport in the body.

9. Amino Acids Profile (Per 100g)	• Non-Essential Amino
• **Essential Amino Acids:**	Acids:
○ **Histidine:** ~0.4g	○ **Alanine:** ~0.6g
○ **Isoleucine:** ~0.9g	○ **Aspartic Acid:** ~1.1g
○ **Leucine:** ~1.4g	○ **Glutamic Acid:** ~2.0g
○ **Lysine:** ~1.5g	○ **Serine:** ~0.5g
○ **Methionine:** ~0.4g	○ **Glycine:** ~0.5g
○ **Phenylalanine:** ~0.7g	○ **Proline:** ~0.4g
○ **Threonine:** ~0.8g	○ **Tyrosine:** ~0.3g
○ **Tryptophan:** ~0.2g	○ **Cysteine:** ~0.2g
○ **Valine:** ~0.9g	
○ **Arginine:** ~0.8g	

Star Baim

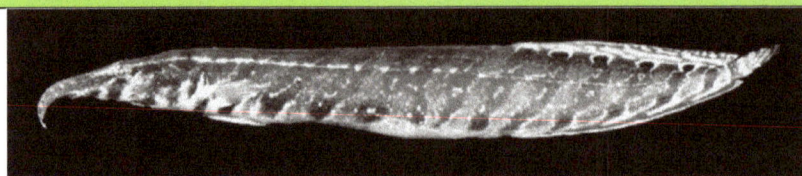

Nutritional Profile of Macrognathus aculeatus

Common Name: Zig-zag Eel, Spiny Eel
Scientific Name: Macrognathus aculeatus

1. Oil Content
- **Category**: Lean
- **Oil Breakdown**: Approximately 2-4% total fat, primarily unsaturated fats.

2. Omega Fatty Acids
- **Omega-3**: About 0.2-0.4g per 100g
  - Supports heart health and reduces inflammation.
- **Omega-6**: Approximately 0.1-0.3g per 100g
  - Important for skin health and cellular functions.
- **Omega-9**: Present in small amounts.

3. Cholesterol Content
- **Cholesterol**: About 40-60 mg per 100g
  - Moderate levels; generally acceptable for most diets.

4. Sodium Content
- **Sodium**: Approximately 30-50 mg per 100g
  - Low sodium content; beneficial for blood pressure management.

5. Mercury Contamination
- **Mercury Levels**: Low
  - Generally safe for consumption with minimal risk of mercury contamination.

6. Nutritional Information (Per 100g)
- **Calories**: ~90-110 kcal
- **Protein**: ~18-20g
  - High protein content supports muscle growth and repair.
- **Fat**: ~2-4g

o   **Saturated Fat**: ~0.3-0.5g
o   **Monounsaturated Fat**: ~0.3-0.5g
o   **Polyunsaturated Fat**: ~0.5-0.7g

7. Vitamins

- **Vitamin B12**: Moderate (~2-3μg)
  o   Essential for nerve function and red blood cell production.
- **Vitamin D**: Present in small amounts
  o   Important for bone health and calcium absorption.
- **Vitamin B6**: Present (~0.2-0.4mg)
  o   Important for amino acid metabolism.

8. Minerals

- **Selenium**: Moderate (~20-30μg)
  o   Acts as an antioxidant, supporting immune health.
- **Phosphorus**: Moderate (~150-200mg)
  o   Crucial for bone health and energy metabolism.
- **Potassium**: Moderate (~200-250mg)
  o   Aids in maintaining fluid balance and regulating blood pressure.
- **Iron**: Present (~0.7-1.0mg)
  o   Important for oxygen transport in the body.

9. Amino Acids Profile (Per 100g)	• Non-Essential Amino Acids:
• **Essential Amino Acids:**	o **Alanine**: ~0.6g
o **Histidine**: ~0.3g	o **Aspartic Acid**: ~1.2g
o **Isoleucine**: ~0.8g	o **Glutamic Acid**: ~2.0g
o **Leucine**: ~1.3g	o **Serine**: ~0.5g
o **Lysine**: ~1.6g	o **Glycine**: ~0.5g
o **Methionine**: ~0.3g	o **Proline**: ~0.4g
o **Phenylalanine**: ~0.7g	o **Tyrosine**: ~0.3g
o **Threonine**: ~0.7g	o **Cysteine**: ~0.2g
o **Tryptophan**: ~0.2g	
o **Valine**: ~0.9g	
o **Arginine**: ~0.9g	

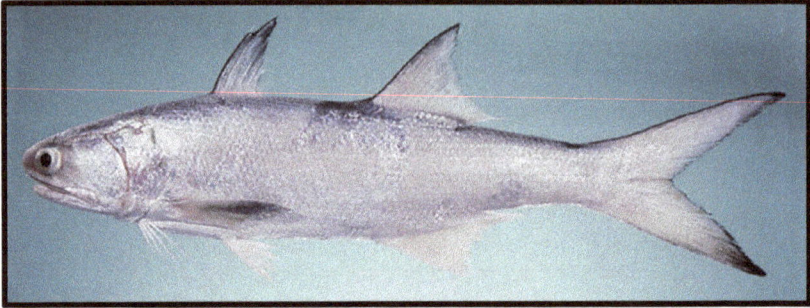

Nutritional Profile of Eleutheronema tetradactylum

Common Name: Fourfinger Threadfin   **Scientific Name**: Eleutheronema tetradactylum

1. Oil Content
- **Category**: Medium-fat
- **Oil Breakdown**: Approximately 5-10% total fat, primarily unsaturated fats.

2. Omega Fatty Acids
- **Omega-3**: About 0.5-0.8g per 100g
  - Supports heart health and reduces inflammation.
- **Omega-6**: Approximately 0.3-0.5g per 100g
  - Important for skin health and cellular functions.
- **Omega-9**: Present in moderate amounts.

3. Cholesterol Content
- **Cholesterol**: About 60-80 mg per 100g
  - Moderate levels; generally acceptable for most diets.

4. Sodium Content
- **Sodium**: Approximately 50-70 mg per 100g
  - Low sodium content; beneficial for blood pressure management.

5. Mercury Contamination
- **Mercury Levels**: Moderate
  - Generally safe for consumption but should be limited for pregnant women and young children.

6. Nutritional Information (Per 100g)
- Calories: ~120-140 kcal
- Protein: ~18-20g
  - High protein content supports muscle growth and repair.
- Fat: ~5-10g
  - Saturated Fat: ~1.0-1.5g
  - Monounsaturated Fat: ~1.5-2.5g
  - Polyunsaturated Fat: ~2.0-3.0g

7. Vitamins
- Vitamin B12: Moderate (~3-4µg)
  - Essential for nerve function and red blood cell production.
- Vitamin D: Moderate (~5-10 IU)
  - Important for bone health and calcium absorption.
- Vitamin B6: Present (~0.3-0.5mg)
  - Important for amino acid metabolism.

8. Minerals
- Selenium: Moderate (~25-35µg)
  - Acts as an antioxidant, supporting immune health.
- Phosphorus: Moderate (~180-220mg)
  - Crucial for bone health and energy metabolism.
- Potassium: Moderate (~250-300mg)
  - Aids in maintaining fluid balance and regulating blood pressure.
- Iron: Present (~0.8-1.2mg)
  - Important for oxygen transport in the body.

9. Amino Acids Profile (Per 100g)	Non-Essential Amino Acids:
Essential Amino Acids:	
○ Histidine: ~0.4g	○ Alanine: ~0.7g
○ Isoleucine: ~0.9g	○ Aspartic Acid: ~1.4g
○ Leucine: ~1.5g	○ Glutamic Acid: ~2.3g
○ Lysine: ~1.8g	○ Serine: ~0.6g
○ Methionine: ~0.4g	○ Glycine: ~0.6g
○ Phenylalanine: ~0.8g	○ Proline: ~0.5g
○ Threonine: ~0.8g	○ Tyrosine: ~0.4g
○ Tryptophan: ~0.2g	○ Cysteine: ~0.3g
○ Valine: ~1.0g	
○ Arginine: ~1.0g	

Taki

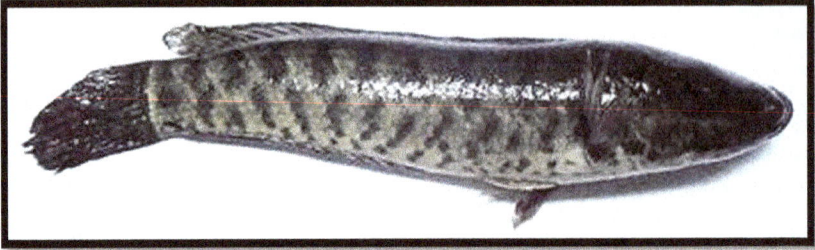

Nutritional Profile of Channa Punctatus

Common Name: Spotted Snakehead
Scientific Name: Channa punctatus

1. Oil Content
- **Category**: Moderate
- **Oil Breakdown**: Approximately 5-10% total fat, primarily unsaturated fats.

2. Omega Fatty Acids
- **Omega-3**: About 0.5-1.0g per 100g
  - Supports cardiovascular health and reduces inflammation.
- **Omega-6**: Approximately 1.0-1.5g per 100g
  - Important for skin health and cellular functions.
- **Omega-9**: Present in smaller amounts.

3. Cholesterol Content
- **Cholesterol**: About 60-80 mg per 100g
  - Moderate levels; generally acceptable for most diets.

4. Sodium Content
- **Sodium**: Approximately 40-60 mg per 100g
  - Low sodium content; beneficial for blood pressure management.

5. Mercury Contamination
- **Mercury Levels**: Generally low
  - Safe for regular consumption.

6. Nutritional Information (Per 100g)
- **Calories**: ~120-140 kcal
- **Protein**: ~18-20g

- o   High protein content supports muscle growth and repair.
- **Fat**: ~5-10g
  - o   **Saturated Fat**: ~1-2g
  - o   **Monounsaturated Fat**: ~1-3g
  - o   **Polyunsaturated Fat**: ~2-4g

7. Vitamins

- **Vitamin B12**: Moderate (~2-3µg)
  - o   Essential for nerve function and red blood cell production.
- **Vitamin D**: Present in small amounts
  - o   Important for bone health and calcium absorption.
- **Vitamin B6**: Present (~0.4-0.5mg)
  - o   Important for amino acid metabolism.

8. Minerals

- **Selenium**: Moderate (~20-25µg)
  - o   Acts as an antioxidant, supporting immune health.
- **Phosphorus**: Moderate (~150-200mg)
  - o   Crucial for bone health and energy metabolism.
- **Potassium**: Moderate (~250-300mg)
  - o   Aids in maintaining fluid balance and regulating blood pressure.
- **Iron**: Present (~1-1.5mg)
  - o   Important for oxygen transport in the body.

9. Amino Acids Profile (Per 100g)	Non-Essential Amino Acids:
Essential Amino Acids:	• **Non-Essential Amino Acids:**
o **Histidine**: ~0.5g	o **Alanine**: ~0.6g
o **Isoleucine**: ~1.0g	o **Aspartic Acid**: ~1.2g
o **Leucine**: ~1.5g	o **Glutamic Acid**: ~2.5g
o **Lysine**: ~2.0g	o **Serine**: ~0.5g
o **Methionine**: ~0.5g	o **Glycine**: ~0.5g
o **Phenylalanine**: ~0.8g	o **Proline**: ~0.3g
o **Threonine**: ~0.9g	o **Tyrosine**: ~0.4g
o **Tryptophan**: ~0.3g	o **Cysteine**: ~0.2g
o **Valine**: ~1.0g	
o **Arginine**: ~1.0g	

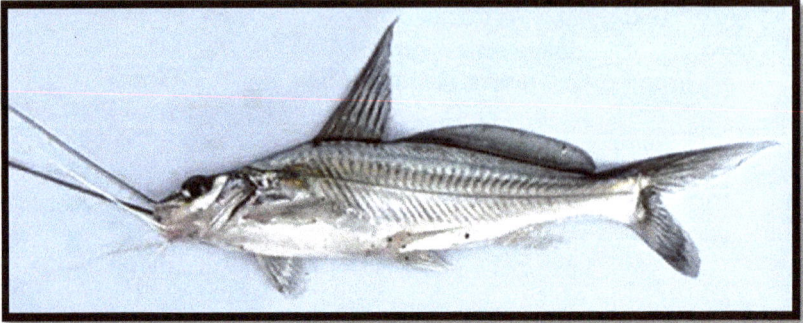

Tengra

Nutritional Profile of Mystus Tengara

Common Name: Tengra Catfish
Scientific Name: Mystus tengara

1. Oil Content
- **Category**: Moderate
- **Oil Breakdown**: Approximately 5-8% total fat, primarily unsaturated fats.

2. Omega Fatty Acids
- **Omega-3**: About 0.5-1.0g per 100g
  - Supports cardiovascular health and reduces inflammation.
- **Omega-6**: Approximately 1.0-1.5g per 100g
  - Important for skin health and cellular functions.
- **Omega-9**: Present in smaller amounts.

3. Cholesterol Content
- **Cholesterol**: About 50-70 mg per 100g
  - Moderate levels; generally acceptable for most diets.

4. Sodium Content
- **Sodium**: Approximately 40-60 mg per 100g
  - Low sodium content; beneficial for blood pressure management.

5. Mercury Contamination
- **Mercury Levels**: Generally low
  - Safe for regular consumption.

6. Nutritional Information (Per 100g)

- **Calories**: ~110-130 kcal
- **Protein**: ~18-20g
  - High protein content supports muscle growth and repair.
- **Fat**: ~5-8g
  - **Saturated Fat**: ~1-2g
  - **Monounsaturated Fat**: ~1-2g
  - **Polyunsaturated Fat**: ~2-4g

7. Vitamins

- **Vitamin B12**: Moderate (~2-3μg)
  - Essential for nerve function and red blood cell production.
- **Vitamin D**: Present in small amounts
  - Important for bone health and calcium absorption.
- **Vitamin B6**: Present (~0.4-0.5mg)
  - Important for amino acid metabolism.

8. Minerals

- **Selenium**: Moderate (~20-25μg)
  - Acts as an antioxidant, supporting immune health.
- **Phosphorus**: Moderate (~150mg)
  - Crucial for bone health and energy metabolism.
- **Potassium**: Moderate (~250-300mg)
  - Aids in maintaining fluid balance and regulating blood pressure.
- **Iron**: Present (~1-1.5mg)
  - Important for oxygen transport in the body.

9. Amino Acids Profile (Per 100g)

- **Essential Amino Acids:**
  - **Histidine**: ~0.5g
  - **Isoleucine**: ~1.0g
  - **Leucine**: ~1.4g
  - **Lysine**: ~2.2g
  - **Methionine**: ~0.5g
  - **Phenylalanine**: ~0.8g
  - **Threonine**: ~0.9g
  - **Tryptophan**: ~0.3g
  - **Valine**: ~1.1g
  - **Arginine**: ~1.0g
- **Non-Essential Amino Acids:**
  - **Alanine**: ~0.7g
  - **Aspartic Acid**: ~1.3g
  - **Glutamic Acid**: ~2.6g
  - **Serine**: ~0.6g
  - **Glycine**: ~0.5g
  - **Proline**: ~0.4g
  - **Tyrosine**: ~0.5g
  - **Cysteine**: ~0.3g

Tengra (Striped)

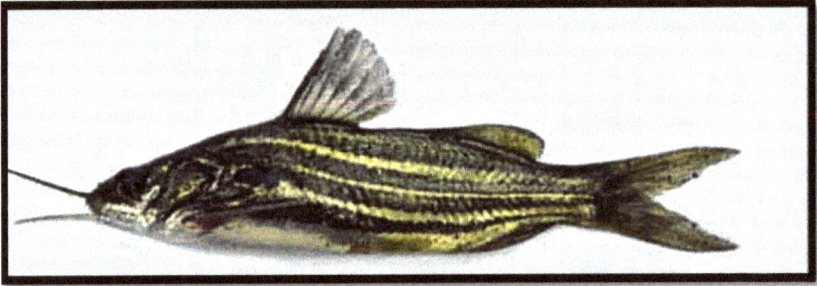

Nutritional Profile of Mystus Vittatus

Common Name: Bojori Catfish
Scientific Name: Mystus vittatus

1. Oil Content
- **Category**: Moderate
- **Oil Breakdown**: Approximately 5-8% total fat, primarily unsaturated fats.

2. Omega Fatty Acids
- **Omega-3**: About 0.5-1.0g per 100g
  - Supports cardiovascular health and reduces inflammation.
- **Omega-6**: Approximately 1.0-1.5g per 100g
  - Important for skin health and cellular functions.
- **Omega-9**: Present in smaller amounts.

3. Cholesterol Content
- **Cholesterol**: About 50-70 mg per 100g
  - Moderate levels; generally acceptable for most diets.

4. Sodium Content
- **Sodium**: Approximately 40-60 mg per 100g
  - Low sodium content; beneficial for blood pressure management.

5. Mercury Contamination
- **Mercury Levels**: Generally low
  - Safe for regular consumption.

6. Nutritional Information (Per 100g)

- **Calories**: ~110-130 kcal
- **Protein**: ~18-20g
  - High protein content supports muscle growth and repair.
- **Fat**: ~5-8g
  - **Saturated Fat**: ~1-2g
  - **Monounsaturated Fat**: ~1-2g
  - **Polyunsaturated Fat**: ~2-4g

7. Vitamins

- **Vitamin B12**: Moderate (~2-3μg)
  - Essential for nerve function and red blood cell production.
- **Vitamin D**: Present in small amounts
  - Important for bone health and calcium absorption.
- **Vitamin B6**: Present (~0.4-0.5mg)
  - Important for amino acid metabolism.

8. Minerals

- **Selenium**: Moderate (~20-25μg)
  - Acts as an antioxidant, supporting immune health.
- **Phosphorus**: Moderate (~150mg)
  - Crucial for bone health and energy metabolism.
- **Potassium**: Moderate (~250-300mg)
  - Aids in maintaining fluid balance and regulating blood pressure.
- **Iron**: Present (~1-1.5mg)
  - Important for oxygen transport in the body.

9. Amino Acids Profile (Per 100g)	Non-Essential Amino Acids:
Essential Amino Acids:	**Non-Essential Amino Acids:**
○ **Histidine**: ~0.5g	○ **Alanine**: ~0.7g
○ **Isoleucine**: ~1.0g	○ **Aspartic Acid**: ~1.3g
○ **Leucine**: ~1.5g	○ **Glutamic Acid**: ~2.6g
○ **Lysine**: ~2.2g	○ **Serine**: ~0.6g
○ **Methionine**: ~0.5g	○ **Glycine**: ~0.5g
○ **Phenylalanine**: ~0.8g	○ **Proline**: ~0.4g
○ **Threonine**: ~0.9g	○ **Tyrosine**: ~0.5g
○ **Tryptophan**: ~0.3g	○ **Cysteine**: ~0.3g
○ **Valine**: ~1.1g	
○ **Arginine**: ~1.0g	

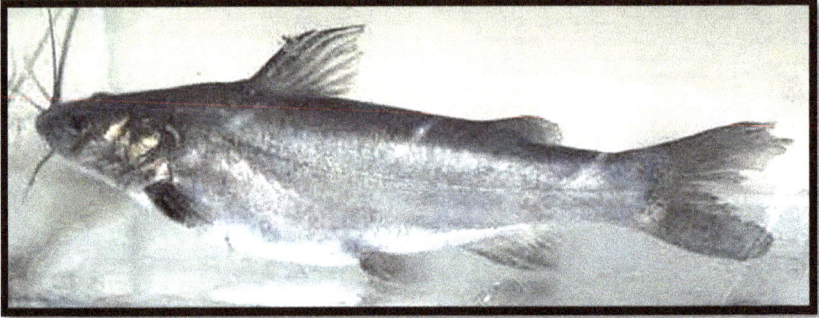

Tengra, Gulsha

Nutritional Profile of Mystus Gulio

Common Name: Gulsha Catfish   **Scientific Name**: Mystus gulio

1. Oil Content
- **Category**: Moderate
- **Oil Breakdown**: Approximately 5-8% total fat, primarily unsaturated fats.

2. Omega Fatty Acids
- **Omega-3**: About 0.5-1.0g per 100g
  - Supports cardiovascular health and reduces inflammation.
- **Omega-6**: Approximately 1.0-1.5g per 100g
  - Important for skin health and cellular functions.
- **Omega-9**: Present in smaller amounts.

3. Cholesterol Content
- **Cholesterol**: About 60-80 mg per 100g
  - Moderate levels; generally acceptable for most diets.

4. Sodium Content
- **Sodium**: Approximately 50-70 mg per 100g
  - Low sodium content; beneficial for blood pressure management.

5. Mercury Contamination
- **Mercury Levels**: Generally low
  - Safe for regular consumption.

6. Nutritional Information (Per 100g)
- Calories: ~120-140 kcal
- Protein: ~18-20g
  - High protein content supports muscle growth and repair.
- Fat: ~5-8g
  - Saturated Fat: ~1-2g
  - Monounsaturated Fat: ~1-3g
  - Polyunsaturated Fat: ~2-4g

7. Vitamins
- Vitamin B12: Moderate (~2-3µg)
  - Essential for nerve function and red blood cell production.
- Vitamin D: Present in small amounts
  - Important for bone health and calcium absorption.
- Vitamin B6: Present (~0.4-0.5mg)
  - Important for amino acid metabolism.

8. Minerals
- Selenium: Moderate (~20-25µg)
  - Acts as an antioxidant, supporting immune health.
- Phosphorus: Moderate (~150mg)
  - Crucial for bone health and energy metabolism.
- Potassium: Moderate (~250-300mg)
  - Aids in maintaining fluid balance and regulating blood pressure.
- Iron: Present (~1-1.5mg)
  - Important for oxygen transport in the body.

9. Amino Acids Profile (Per 100g)	Non-Essential Amino Acids:
Essential Amino Acids:	
o Histidine: ~0.5g	o Alanine: ~0.6g
o Isoleucine: ~1.0g	o Aspartic Acid: ~1.2g
o Leucine: ~1.4g	o Glutamic Acid: ~2.5g
o Lysine: ~2.0g	o Serine: ~0.5g
o Methionine: ~0.5g	o Glycine: ~0.5g
o Phenylalanine: ~0.8g	o Proline: ~0.4g
o Threonine: ~0.9g	o Tyrosine: ~0.5g
o Tryptophan: ~0.3g	o Cysteine: ~0.2g
o Valine: ~1.1g	
o Arginine: ~1.0g	

Tilapia

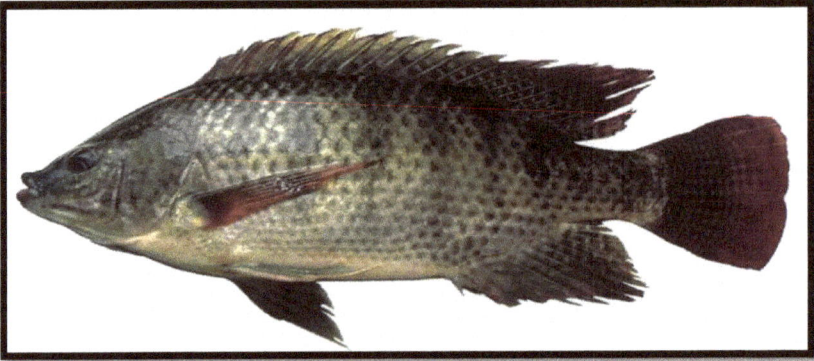

Nutritional Profile of Oreochromis niloticus

Common Name: Nile Tilapia
Scientific Name: Oreochromis niloticus

1. Oil Content
- **Category**: Lean to Moderate
- **Oil Breakdown**: Approximately 2-5% total fat, with a balance of saturated and unsaturated fats.

2. Omega Fatty Acids
- **Omega-3**: About 0.2-0.5g per 100g
  - Supports heart health and reduces inflammation.
- **Omega-6**: Approximately 1.5-3.0g per 100g
  - Important for skin health and cellular functions.
- **Omega-9**: Present in smaller amounts.

3. Cholesterol Content
- **Cholesterol**: About 50-60 mg per 100g
  - Moderate levels; generally acceptable for most diets.

4. Sodium Content
- **Sodium**: Approximately 60-80 mg per 100g
  - Low sodium content; beneficial for blood pressure management.

5. Mercury Contamination
- **Mercury Levels**: Generally low
  - Safe for regular consumption.

6. Nutritional Information (Per 100g)
- Calories: ~120-130 kcal
- Protein: ~20-22g
  - High protein content supports muscle growth and repair.
- Fat: ~2-5g
  - **Saturated Fat**: ~0.5-1g
  - **Monounsaturated Fat**: ~1-2g
  - **Polyunsaturated Fat**: ~1-2g

7. Vitamins
- **Vitamin B12**: Moderate (~2-3µg)
  - Essential for nerve function and red blood cell production.
- **Vitamin D**: Present in small amounts
  - Important for bone health and calcium absorption.
- **Vitamin B6**: Present (~0.5mg)
  - Important for amino acid metabolism.

8. Minerals
- **Selenium**: Moderate (~20-30µg)
  - Acts as an antioxidant, supporting immune health.
- **Phosphorus**: Moderate (~150mg)
  - Crucial for bone health and energy metabolism.
- **Potassium**: Moderate (~300mg)
  - Aids in maintaining fluid balance and regulating blood pressure.
- **Iron**: Present (~0.8-1.0mg)
  - Important for oxygen transport in the body.

9. Amino Acids Profile (Per 100g)	
Essential Amino Acids:	• **Non-Essential Amino Acids:**
○ **Histidine**: ~0.5g	○ **Alanine**: ~0.8g
○ **Isoleucine**: ~1.0g	○ **Aspartic Acid**: ~1.4g
○ **Leucine**: ~1.6g	○ **Glutamic Acid**: ~2.7g
○ **Lysine**: ~2.4g	○ **Serine**: ~0.7g
○ **Methionine**: ~0.5g	○ **Glycine**: ~0.5g
○ **Phenylalanine**: ~0.9g	○ **Proline**: ~0.4g
○ **Threonine**: ~0.9g	○ **Tyrosine**: ~0.5g
○ **Tryptophan**: ~0.2g	○ **Cysteine**: ~0.3g
○ **Valine**: ~1.1g	
○ **Arginine**: ~1.1g	

Trout (Rainbow)

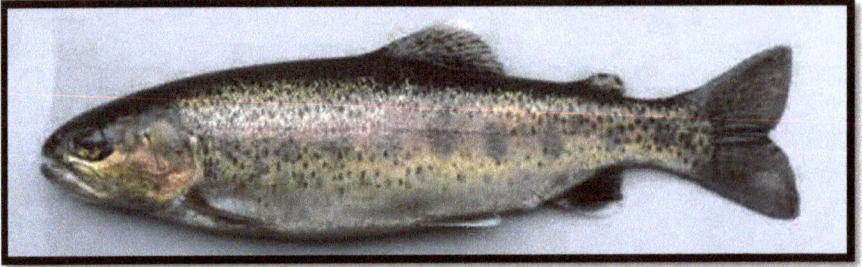

Nutritional Profile of Oncorhynchus mykiss

Common Name: Rainbow Trout
Scientific Name: Oncorhynchus mykiss

1. Oil Content
- **Category**: Fatty
- **Oil Breakdown**: Approximately 6-12% total fat, primarily unsaturated fats.

2. Omega Fatty Acids
- **Omega-3**: About 1.0-2.5g per 100g
  - Supports heart health and reduces inflammation.
- **Omega-6**: Approximately 0.5-1.0g per 100g
  - Important for skin health and cellular functions.
- **Omega-9**: Present in moderate amounts.

3. Cholesterol Content
- **Cholesterol**: About 60-70 mg per 100g
  - Moderate levels; generally acceptable for most diets.

4. Sodium Content
- **Sodium**: Approximately 50-60 mg per 100g
  - Low sodium content; beneficial for blood pressure management.

5. Mercury Contamination
- **Mercury Levels**: Generally low
  - Safe for regular consumption.

6. Nutritional Information (Per 100g)
- **Calories**: ~140-170 kcal

- **Protein**: ~20-22g
  - High protein content supports muscle growth and repair.
- **Fat**: ~6-12g
  - **Saturated Fat**: ~1-2g
  - **Monounsaturated Fat**: ~2-4g
  - **Polyunsaturated Fat**: ~2-4g

7. Vitamins

- **Vitamin B12**: High (~4-5µg)
  - Essential for nerve function and red blood cell production.
- **Vitamin D**: Present in moderate amounts
  - Important for bone health and calcium absorption.
- **Vitamin B6**: Present (~0.5-1.0mg)
  - Important for amino acid metabolism.

8. Minerals

- **Selenium**: High (~25-30µg)
  - Acts as an antioxidant, supporting immune health.
- **Phosphorus**: Moderate (~200mg)
  - Crucial for bone health and energy metabolism.
- **Potassium**: Moderate (~300-400mg)
  - Aids in maintaining fluid balance and regulating blood pressure.
- **Iron**: Present (~1-1.5mg)
  - Important for oxygen transport in the body.

9. Amino Acids Profile (Per 100g)	Non-Essential Amino Acids:
Essential Amino Acids:	
○ **Histidine**: ~0.5g	○ **Alanine**: ~0.8g
○ **Isoleucine**: ~1.0g	○ **Aspartic Acid**: ~1.5g
○ **Leucine**: ~1.5g	○ **Glutamic Acid**: ~3.0g
○ **Lysine**: ~2.3g	○ **Serine**: ~0.7g
○ **Methionine**: ~0.5g	○ **Glycine**: ~0.6g
○ **Phenylalanine**: ~0.8g	○ **Proline**: ~0.5g
○ **Threonine**: ~0.9g	○ **Tyrosine**: ~0.5g
○ **Tryptophan**: ~0.2g	○ **Cysteine**: ~0.3g
○ **Valine**: ~1.1g	
○ **Arginine**: ~1.0g	

Tuna (Skipjack)

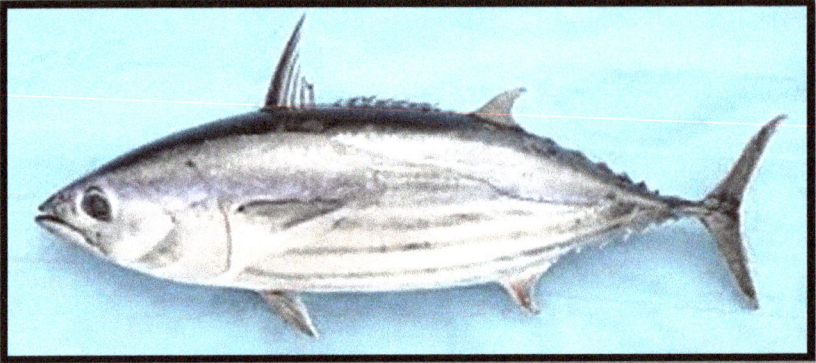

Nutritional Profile of Katsuwonus pelamis

Common Name: Skipjack Tuna
Scientific Name: Katsuwonus pelamis

1. Oil Content
- **Category**: Fatty
- **Oil Breakdown**: Approximately 10-15% total fat, primarily unsaturated fats.

2. Omega Fatty Acids
- **Omega-3**: About 1.0-2.5g per 100g
  - Supports heart health and reduces inflammation.
- **Omega-6**: Approximately 0.4-1.0g per 100g
  - Important for skin health and cellular functions.
- **Omega-9**: Present in moderate amounts.

3. Cholesterol Content
- **Cholesterol**: About 50-70 mg per 100g
  - Moderate levels; generally acceptable for most diets.

4. Sodium Content
- **Sodium**: Approximately 60-70 mg per 100g
  - Low sodium content; beneficial for blood pressure management.

5. Mercury Contamination
- **Mercury Levels**: Moderate

o Caution advised with high consumption; lower levels in smaller fish.

6. Nutritional Information (Per 100g)
- **Calories**: ~140-170 kcal
- **Protein**: ~23-25g
    o High protein content supports muscle growth and repair.
- **Fat**: ~10-15g
    o **Saturated Fat**: ~2-3g
    o **Monounsaturated Fat**: ~3-4g
    o **Polyunsaturated Fat**: ~4-5g

7. Vitamins
- **Vitamin B12**: High (~3-4µg)
    o Essential for nerve function and red blood cell production.
- **Vitamin D**: Present in moderate amounts
    o Important for bone health and calcium absorption.
- **Vitamin B6**: Present (~0.5-0.8mg)
    o Important for amino acid metabolism.

8. Minerals
- **Selenium**: High (~30-40µg)
    o Acts as an antioxidant, supporting immune health.
- **Phosphorus**: Moderate (~200mg)
    o Crucial for bone health and energy metabolism.
- **Potassium**: Moderate (~350-400mg)
    o Aids in maintaining fluid balance and regulating blood pressure.
- **Iron**: Present (~1-1.5mg)
    o Important for oxygen transport in the body.

9. Amino Acids Profile (Per 100g)	Non-Essential
Essential Amino Acids:	**Amino Acids**:
o **Histidine**: ~0.5g	o **Alanine**: ~0.9g
o **Isoleucine**: ~1.0g	o **Aspartic Acid**: ~1.8g
o **Leucine**: ~1.6g	o **Glutamic Acid**: ~3.2g
o **Lysine**: ~2.5g	o **Serine**: ~0.8g
o **Methionine**: ~0.5g	o **Glycine**: ~0.5g
o **Phenylalanine**: ~1.0g	o **Proline**: ~0.6g
o **Threonine**: ~0.9g	o **Tyrosine**: ~0.4g
o **Tryptophan**: ~0.3g	o **Cysteine**: ~0.2g
o **Valine**: ~1.2g	
o **Arginine**: ~1.2g	

Tuna (Yellowfin)

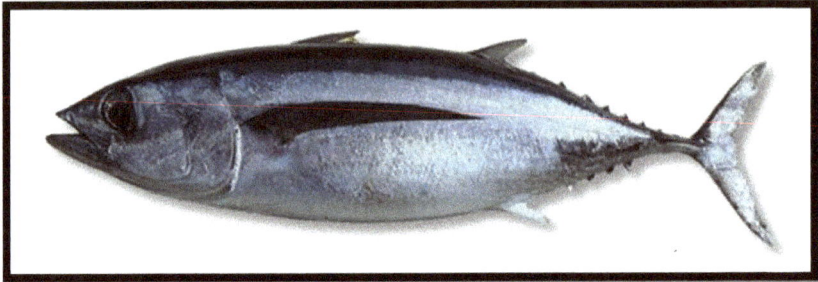

Nutritional Profile of Thunnus albacares

Common Name: Yellowfin Tuna
Scientific Name: Thunnus albacares

1. Oil Content
- **Category**: Fatty
- **Oil Breakdown**: Approximately 10-20% total fat, primarily unsaturated fats.

2. Omega Fatty Acids
- **Omega-3**: About 1.5-2.5g per 100g
  - Supports heart health and reduces inflammation.
- **Omega-6**: Approximately 0.5-1.0g per 100g
  - Important for skin health and cellular functions.
- **Omega-9**: Present in moderate amounts.

3. Cholesterol Content
- **Cholesterol**: About 60-70 mg per 100g
  - Moderate levels; generally acceptable for most diets.

4. Sodium Content
- **Sodium**: Approximately 50-70 mg per 100g
  - Low sodium content; beneficial for blood pressure management.

5. Mercury Contamination
- **Mercury Levels**: Moderate to high
  - Caution advised with high consumption; larger fish tend to accumulate more mercury.

6. Nutritional Information (Per 100g)
- **Calories**: ~130-180 kcal

- **Protein**: ~24-26g
  - High protein content supports muscle growth and repair.
- **Fat**: ~10-20g
  - **Saturated Fat**: ~2-4g
  - **Monounsaturated Fat**: ~3-5g
  - **Polyunsaturated Fat**: ~3-6g

7. Vitamins

- **Vitamin B12**: High (~4-5μg)
  - Essential for nerve function and red blood cell production.
- **Vitamin D**: Present in moderate amounts
  - Important for bone health and calcium absorption.
- **Vitamin B6**: Present (~0.5-1.0mg)
  - Important for amino acid metabolism.

8. Minerals

- **Selenium**: High (~30-40μg)
  - Acts as an antioxidant, supporting immune health.
- **Phosphorus**: Moderate (~200mg)
  - Crucial for bone health and energy metabolism.
- **Potassium**: Moderate (~350-400mg)
  - Aids in maintaining fluid balance and regulating blood pressure.
- **Iron**: Present (~1-1.5mg)
  - Important for oxygen transport in the body.

9. Amino Acids Profile (Per 100g)	Non-Essential Amino Acids:
Essential Amino Acids:	
○ **Histidine**: ~0.5g	○ **Alanine**: ~0.8g
○ **Isoleucine**: ~1.0g	○ **Aspartic Acid**: ~1.6g
○ **Leucine**: ~1.6g	○ **Glutamic Acid**: ~3.1g
○ **Lysine**: ~2.4g	○ **Serine**: ~0.7g
○ **Methionine**: ~0.6g	○ **Glycine**: ~0.5g
○ **Phenylalanine**: ~0.9g	○ **Proline**: ~0.5g
○ **Threonine**: ~0.9g	○ **Tyrosine**: ~0.4g
○ **Tryptophan**: ~0.2g	○ **Cysteine**: ~0.3g
○ **Valine**: ~1.1g	
○ **Arginine**: ~1.2g	

Please note these figures have been collated from various sources that were conducted at various times by different groups and labs. These are for reference guide and are not any medical guidelines. All readers to take reference and do their own due-diligences.

Essential Amino Acids and Their Health Benefits

1. **Histidine**
   - **Benefits**: Important for growth and repair of tissues, production of blood cells, and maintaining nerve cells' protective myelin sheaths. Acts as a precursor to histamine, crucial for immune response, digestion, and sexual function.
2. **Isoleucine**
   - **Benefits**: Aids in muscle metabolism and is heavily concentrated in muscle tissue. Important for immune function, hemoglobin production, and energy regulation.
3. **Leucine**
   - **Benefits**: Stimulates muscle protein synthesis, aids in muscle repair and growth, regulates blood sugar levels, and promotes the healing of bones, skin, and muscle tissues.
4. **Lysine**
   - **Benefits**: Crucial for protein synthesis, hormone and enzyme production, calcium absorption, and immune function. It helps in collagen formation and tissue repair.
5. **Methionine**
   - **Benefits**: Acts as an antioxidant, assists in the breakdown of fats, and helps in detoxifying harmful substances. It's also essential for healthy skin, hair, and nail growth.
6. **Phenylalanine**
   - **Benefits**: Precursor to neurotransmitters like dopamine, norepinephrine, and epinephrine, which are important for mood regulation and cognitive functions. It also plays a role in the structure and function of proteins and enzymes.
7. **Threonine**
   - **Benefits**: Crucial for the formation of collagen and elastin, which are important for skin and connective tissues. It also supports immune function and fat metabolism.
8. **Tryptophan**
   - **Benefits**: Precursor to serotonin, which regulates mood, sleep, and appetite. It also helps in the production of melatonin, which is vital for sleep regulation.

9. **Valine**
   - o **Benefits**: Stimulates muscle growth and regeneration, plays a role in energy production, and helps repair tissues. It's also important for cognitive function and immune response.
10. **Arginine**
   - o **Benefits**: Precursor to nitric oxide, which helps relax blood vessels and improve circulation. It plays a role in wound healing, hormone release, and immune function.

Non-Essential Amino Acids and Their Health Benefits
1. **Alanine**
   - o **Benefits**: Involved in the metabolism of glucose and is critical for energy production. It helps maintain blood sugar levels and supports the immune system.
2. **Aspartic Acid**
   - o **Benefits**: Plays a role in hormone production and release, and is involved in the function of the nervous system. It's also important for energy production.
3. **Glutamic Acid**
   - o **Benefits**: Acts as a neurotransmitter and is crucial for brain function. It is also involved in the metabolism of amino acids and the detoxification of ammonia.
4. **Serine**
   - o **Benefits**: Important for the synthesis of proteins, enzymes, and neurotransmitters. It supports immune function and muscle growth.
5. **Glycine**
   - o **Benefits**: Crucial for the production of collagen, which is important for skin, joints, and connective tissues. It also supports the central nervous system and digestive health.
6. **Proline**
   - o **Benefits**: Essential for the production of collagen, which is vital for skin elasticity and wound healing. It also helps maintain and repair muscles and joints.
7. **Tyrosine**
   - o **Benefits**: Precursor to neurotransmitters like dopamine, norepinephrine, and epinephrine, which are important for mood, alertness, and stress response.
8. **Cysteine**
   - o **Benefits**: Supports the production of the antioxidant glutathione, which helps protect cells from damage. It's also important for skin health and detoxification processes.

Health Conditions Remedied by Specific Amino Acids

1. **Histidine**
   - Conditions:
     - **Arthritis**: Histidine has anti-inflammatory properties that can help alleviate symptoms of arthritis.
     - **Allergies**: As a precursor to histamine, it can modulate allergic responses.
2. **Isoleucine**
   - Conditions:
     - **Muscle Wasting Diseases**: Helps prevent muscle breakdown in conditions like sarcopenia and cachexia.
     - **Diabetes**: Regulates blood sugar and supports energy metabolism.
3. **Leucine**
   - Conditions:
     - **Muscle Atrophy**: Stimulates muscle protein synthesis, important for conditions like muscular dystrophy.
     - **Obesity**: Regulates appetite and supports fat loss.
4. **Lysine**
   - Conditions:
     - **Cold Sores (Herpes Simplex Virus)**: Reduces the frequency and severity of outbreaks.
     - **Osteoporosis**: Enhances calcium absorption, important for bone health.
5. **Methionine**
   - Conditions:
     - **Liver Disease**: Detoxifies harmful substances and prevents fat buildup in the liver.
     - **Chronic Fatigue Syndrome**: Supports energy production and metabolism.
6. **Phenylalanine**
   - Conditions:
     - **Depression**: As a precursor to neurotransmitters, it can improve mood and alleviate depression.
     - **Chronic Pain**: Phenylalanine can increase endorphin levels, providing pain relief.
7. **Threonine**
   - Conditions:
     - **Multiple Sclerosis**: Supports the production of myelin, the protective sheath around nerves.

- **Digestive Disorders**: Promotes gut health by supporting mucus production in the digestive tract.

8. **Tryptophan**
   o **Conditions**:
     - **Insomnia**: As a precursor to serotonin and melatonin, it helps regulate sleep.
     - **Anxiety and Depression**: Improves mood and alleviates symptoms of anxiety and depression.

9. **Valine**
   o **Conditions**:
     - **Muscle Recovery**: Helps repair muscle tissue after exercise or injury.
     - **Liver Disease**: Supports liver function and detoxification.

10. **Arginine**
    o **Conditions**:
      - **Cardiovascular Disease**: Improves blood flow and reduces blood pressure.
      - **Erectile Dysfunction**: Enhances blood circulation, important for erectile function.

Non-Essential Amino Acids and Health Conditions

1. **Alanine**
   o **Conditions**:
     - **Hypoglycemia**: Helps maintain blood sugar levels.
     - **Chronic Fatigue Syndrome**: Provides energy and supports metabolism.

2. **Aspartic Acid**
   o **Conditions**:
     - **Chronic Fatigue Syndrome**: Enhances energy production.
     - **Depression**: Supports neurotransmitter production.

3. **Glutamic Acid**
   o **Conditions**:
     - **Neurodegenerative Diseases**: Acts as a neurotransmitter and supports brain function.
     - **Mental Fatigue**: Improves cognitive function and reduces mental exhaustion.

4. **Serine**
   o **Conditions**:
     - **Cognitive Disorders**: Important for brain function and memory.
     - **Autoimmune Diseases**: Supports immune system regulation.

5. **Glycine**

- o Conditions:
  - Insomnia: Improves sleep quality.
  - Joint Pain: Supports collagen production, important for joint health.
6. **Proline**
  - o Conditions:
    - **Skin Disorders**: Promotes collagen formation and wound healing.
    - **Joint Disorders**: Important for maintaining and repairing connective tissues.
7. **Tyrosine**
  - o Conditions:
    - **Hypothyroidism**: Precursor to thyroid hormones.
    - **Stress and Anxiety**: Supports the production of stress-related neurotransmitters.
8. **Cysteine**
  - o Conditions:
    - **Chronic Obstructive Pulmonary Disease (COPD)**: Acts as an antioxidant and reduces mucus.
    - **Detoxification**: Supports the body's detoxification processes and liver health.

Health Conditions Remedied by Minerals Found in Fish

Fish are rich sources of several essential minerals that play vital roles in human health. Here are specific known health conditions that can be remedied or alleviated by minerals commonly found in fish:

1. **Calcium**
- **Conditions:**
  - o **Osteoporosis**: Calcium is crucial for maintaining bone density and preventing osteoporosis.
  - o **Hypertension**: Adequate calcium intake can help maintain healthy blood pressure levels.
  - o **Premenstrual Syndrome (PMS)**: Calcium can reduce symptoms such as bloating, mood swings, and cramps.

2. **Iron**
- **Conditions:**

- o **Iron Deficiency Anemia**: Iron is essential for hemoglobin production and red blood cell formation, preventing and treating anemia.
- o **Fatigue**: Iron enhances energy levels by improving oxygen transport in the blood.
- o **Restless Legs Syndrome (RLS)**: Iron supplementation can alleviate symptoms of RLS, particularly when caused by iron deficiency.

3. **Magnesium**
- **Conditions**:
  - o **Migraines**: Magnesium can reduce the frequency and severity of migraine attacks.
  - o **Type 2 Diabetes**: Magnesium helps improve insulin sensitivity and blood sugar control.
  - o **Muscle Cramps and Spasms**: Magnesium relieves muscle tension and promotes relaxation, beneficial for cramps and spasms.

4. **Phosphorus**
- **Conditions**:
  - o **Bone and Teeth Health**: Phosphorus, in conjunction with calcium, is vital for the development and maintenance of strong bones and teeth.
  - o **Fatigue**: Phosphorus plays a role in energy production and storage.
  - o **Muscle Weakness**: Phosphorus supports muscle function and repair.

5. **Potassium**
- **Conditions**:
  - o **Hypertension**: Potassium helps lower blood pressure by balancing sodium levels.
  - o **Stroke**: Adequate potassium intake reduces the risk of stroke by maintaining cardiovascular health.
  - o **Kidney Stones**: Potassium helps prevent kidney stone formation by reducing calcium excretion.

6. **Selenium**
- **Conditions**:
  - o **Thyroid Disorders**: Selenium is essential for the metabolism and function of thyroid hormones.
  - o **Immune System Support**: Selenium enhances immune response and reduces inflammation.
  - o **Cancer Prevention**: Selenium acts as an antioxidant, reducing the risk of certain cancers.

7. **Zinc**
- **Conditions**:

179

- o **Common Cold**: Zinc can reduce the duration and severity of cold symptoms.
- o **Acne**: Zinc supports skin health and reduces inflammation.
- o **Age-Related Macular Degeneration (AMD)**: Zinc helps slow the progression of vision loss in AMD.

8. Iodine
- Conditions:
  - o **Hypothyroidism**: Iodine is necessary for the production of thyroid hormones.
  - o **Goiter**: Iodine prevents and treats the enlargement of the thyroid gland.
  - o **Cognitive Impairment**: Iodine is essential for brain development and cognitive function.

9. Copper
- Conditions:
  - o **Anemia**: Copper works with iron to form red blood cells, preventing anemia.
  - o **Osteoporosis**: Copper supports bone density and overall bone health.
  - o **Heart Disease**: Copper plays a role in maintaining heart health by supporting blood vessel integrity.

10. Manganese
- Conditions:
  - o **Bone Health**: Manganese contributes to bone formation and metabolism.
  - o **Diabetes**: Manganese aids in glucose metabolism and regulation.
  - o **Wound Healing**: Manganese is essential for collagen formation and skin repair.

Can You Have Too Much Fish?

While fish is a highly nutritious food and an important part of a balanced diet, consuming too much fish can have adverse effects due to potential contaminants and excessive intake of certain nutrients. Here are some considerations regarding the risks of consuming too much fish:

1. Mercury Contamination
- **Risk**: Mercury is a heavy metal that can accumulate in fish, particularly in larger and longer-living species like tuna, swordfish, and shark. High

levels of mercury can cause neurological and developmental problems, particularly in pregnant women, infants, and young children.

- **Recommendation**: Limit consumption of high-mercury fish and choose fish with lower mercury levels such as salmon, sardines, and trout. The FDA and EPA recommend that pregnant women and young children eat 2-3 servings of low-mercury fish per week.

2. Polychlorinated Biphenyls (PCBs) and Dioxins

- **Risk**: PCBs and dioxins are environmental pollutants that can accumulate in fish. These chemicals have been linked to cancer and other health issues.
- **Recommendation**: Consume a variety of fish to minimize exposure to these contaminants and choose fish from less polluted waters when possible.

3. Excessive Intake of Omega-3 Fatty Acids

- **Risk**: While omega-3 fatty acids are beneficial for heart health and inflammation, very high intakes can lead to excessive bleeding, immune system suppression, and potential interactions with medications like blood thinners.
- **Recommendation**: Follow recommended guidelines for fish consumption, which typically suggest 2-3 servings of fatty fish per week to balance benefits and risks.

4. Overconsumption of Sodium

- **Risk**: Some fish, particularly processed or canned varieties, can be high in sodium, which can contribute to high blood pressure and cardiovascular issues.
- **Recommendation**: Choose fresh or frozen fish over canned or smoked varieties to reduce sodium intake. Always check labels for sodium content.

5. Vitamin and Mineral Toxicity

- **Risk**: Consuming too much fish high in certain vitamins and minerals (e.g., vitamin A in liver oils) can lead to toxicity. Excessive vitamin A can cause liver damage, dizziness, nausea, and even death.
- **Recommendation**: Maintain a varied diet to avoid excessive intake of any single nutrient.

Summary and Recommendations

While fish is an excellent source of protein, omega-3 fatty acids, and essential nutrients, it is important to consume it in moderation and make informed choices to avoid potential health risks. Here are some general guidelines:

- **Variety**: Eat a variety of fish to minimize exposure to contaminants and to benefit from different nutrients.
- **Moderation**: Follow dietary guidelines which generally recommend 2-3 servings of fish per week.

- **Low-Mercury Choices**: Opt for fish lower in mercury, such as salmon, sardines, and mackerel, especially for pregnant women, nursing mothers, and young children.
- **Preparation Methods**: Choose fresh, frozen, or low-sodium canned fish, and be mindful of preparation methods to avoid added fats and sodium.
- **Consultation**: If you have specific health concerns or conditions, consult with a healthcare provider or a registered dietitian to tailor fish consumption to your individual needs.

By following these recommendations, you can enjoy the health benefits of fish while minimizing potential risks.

Best Ways to Prepare and Eat Fish for Maximum Health Benefits

To maximize the health benefits of fish while minimizing potential risks, consider the following methods of preparation and consumption:

1. Baking
- **Health Benefits**: Baking is a method that uses dry heat, preserving most of the nutrients in the fish without adding extra fat. It is a heart-healthy option.
- **Tips**: Season with herbs, spices, lemon juice, or a drizzle of olive oil. Wrap the fish in parchment paper or foil to keep it moist and flavorful.

2. Grilling
- **Health Benefits**: Grilling imparts a smoky flavor without the need for added fats. It allows excess fat to drip away from the fish, making it a lower-calorie option.
- **Tips**: Preheat the grill to avoid sticking. Marinate the fish to enhance flavor and moisture. Be cautious to avoid charring, as it can create harmful compounds.

3. Steaming
- **Health Benefits**: Steaming preserves nutrients and natural flavors without the need for oil or fat. It is an excellent method for maintaining the fish's moisture and texture.
- **Tips**: Use a steamer basket or a bamboo steamer. Add aromatic herbs, ginger, or garlic to the steaming water for added flavor.

4. Poaching

- **Health Benefits**: Poaching gently cooks fish in water or broth, maintaining its delicate texture and nutrient profile. This method does not require added fats.
- **Tips**: Use flavorful liquids like vegetable broth, wine, or a mix of water and lemon juice. Keep the liquid at a simmer, not a boil, to avoid overcooking.

5. Sautéing

- **Health Benefits**: Sautéing in a small amount of healthy oil (like olive oil) can create a crispy exterior while keeping the inside moist and tender.
- **Tips**: Use a non-stick pan to reduce the amount of oil needed. Add fresh herbs, garlic, or a squeeze of citrus to enhance the flavor.

6. Broiling

- **Health Benefits**: Broiling uses high heat from above, similar to grilling. It is quick and can give a nice crispy texture without much added fat.
- **Tips**: Place fish on a broiler pan to allow fat to drain away. Watch closely to prevent burning, as broiling is a fast cooking method.

7. Ceviche

- **Health Benefits**: Ceviche "cooks" fish using the acid from citrus juices, preserving nutrients and creating a fresh, light dish. It is often combined with vegetables and herbs.
- **Tips**: Use only very fresh, high-quality fish to minimize the risk of foodborne illness. Marinate in citrus juice (like lime or lemon) and add ingredients like onions, peppers, and cilantro.

Additional Tips for Healthy Fish Consumption

- **Choose Sustainable Options**: Opt for sustainably sourced fish to support environmental health and ensure a supply of healthy fish for the future. Look for certifications from organizations like the Marine Stewardship Council (MSC).
- **Avoid Deep-Frying**: Deep-frying adds unnecessary calories and fat, potentially negating the health benefits of fish.
- **Watch for Mercury**: Choose fish known to have lower mercury levels, especially if you are pregnant, nursing, or feeding young children. Good low-mercury options include salmon, sardines, and trout.
- **Pair with Vegetables**: Complement your fish dishes with a variety of vegetables to create a balanced, nutrient-dense meal.
- **Limit Added Salt**: Use herbs, spices, and citrus instead of salt to enhance flavor without increasing sodium intake.

Oiliest fish known to man

The oiliest fish known to man, often cited for its exceptionally high oil content, is the **Atlantic mackerel (Scomber scombrus)**. This fish is renowned for its rich, oily flesh, which is packed with beneficial omega-3 fatty acids. Here are a few key points about the Atlantic mackerel and other similarly oily fish:

Atlantic Mackerel (Scomber scombrus)
- **Oil Content**: Atlantic mackerel contains approximately 13-15 grams of fat per 100 grams of fish, making it one of the richest sources of fish oil.
- **Omega-3 Fatty Acids**: High in EPA (eicosapentaenoic acid) and DHA (docosahexaenoic acid), which are beneficial for heart health, brain function, and reducing inflammation.
- **Nutritional Profile**: Besides its high-fat content, Atlantic mackerel is also a good source of protein, vitamin B12, vitamin D, selenium, and niacin.

Other Notably Oily Fish
1. **Pacific Saury (Cololabis saira)**
   o **Oil Content**: Approximately 11-12 grams of fat per 100 grams.
   o **Benefits**: Rich in omega-3s and vitamin D.
2. **Herring (Clupea harengus)**
   o **Oil Content**: About 10-18 grams of fat per 100 grams, varying by season and preparation.
   o **Benefits**: Excellent source of omega-3 fatty acids, vitamin D, and selenium.
3. **Salmon (Salmo salar)**
   o **Oil Content**: Approximately 11-13 grams of fat per 100 grams, with variations between wild and farmed.
   o **Benefits**: High in omega-3s, protein, B vitamins, and antioxidants like astaxanthin.
4. **Sardines (Sardinella spp.)**
   o **Oil Content**: Around 10-15 grams of fat per 100 grams.
   o **Benefits**: High in omega-3 fatty acids, calcium (especially when consumed with bones), and vitamin D.
5. **Anchovies (Engraulis spp.)**
   o **Oil Content**: About 9-12 grams of fat per 100 grams.
   o **Benefits**: Rich in omega-3s, calcium, and protein.

Health Benefits of Oily Fish

- **Cardiovascular Health**: Omega-3 fatty acids in oily fish can reduce the risk of heart disease by lowering triglycerides, reducing blood pressure, and improving cholesterol levels.
- **Brain Function**: DHA is crucial for brain health, improving cognitive function, and potentially reducing the risk of neurodegenerative diseases.
- **Anti-inflammatory Properties**: Omega-3s help reduce inflammation, which can benefit conditions like arthritis and other inflammatory diseases.
- **Nutrient-Rich**: Oily fish are packed with vitamins and minerals, such as vitamin D (important for bone health), vitamin B12 (important for nerve function and blood formation), and selenium (an antioxidant that helps protect cells).

Consumption Recommendations

While oily fish provide numerous health benefits, it's important to consume them in moderation due to potential contaminants like mercury and PCBs. The FDA and EPA recommend eating 2-3 servings of low-mercury fish per week, including a variety of species to balance the nutritional benefits and minimize risks.

By incorporating oily fish like Atlantic mackerel, herring, and salmon into your diet, you can reap significant health benefits while enjoying a diverse and flavorful range of seafood options.

Bangladeshi Fish and Diabetes

In Bangladesh, several types of fish are beneficial for managing diabetes due to their high nutritional value and health benefits. Among them, **Hilsa (Tenualosa ilisha)** is often highlighted for its rich content of omega-3 fatty acids, which are known to have anti-inflammatory and cardioprotective properties. However, considering overall accessibility, nutritional content, and local dietary habits, here are some of the best Bangladeshi fish for managing diabetes:

1. Hilsa (Tenualosa ilisha)

Nutritional Profile: Rich in omega-3 fatty acids, high-quality protein, and essential vitamins like vitamin D and B12.

Benefits: Omega-3s improve insulin sensitivity, reduce inflammation, and support heart health. Protein aids in blood sugar regulation.

2. Rohu (Labeo rohita)

Nutritional Profile: High in protein, omega-3 and omega-6 fatty acids, and essential minerals such as iron, zinc, and potassium.

Benefits: Supports cardiovascular health, enhances immune function, and helps maintain stable blood sugar levels due to its high-quality protein content.

3. Catla (Catla catla)

Nutritional Profile: High in protein, omega-3 fatty acids, and essential minerals like calcium and phosphorus.

Benefits: Promotes heart health, bone health, and helps in regulating blood sugar levels.

4. Tilapia (Oreochromis niloticus)

Nutritional Profile: High in protein, low in fat, and contains omega-3 fatty acids, vitamins, and minerals.

Benefits: Supports muscle health, maintains stable blood glucose levels, and provides essential nutrients with low calorie content.

5. Pangasius (Pangasius pangasius)

Nutritional Profile: High in protein and omega-3 fatty acids, and low in saturated fat.

Benefits: Supports heart health, provides essential amino acids, and helps in controlling blood sugar levels.

Specific Benefits for Managing Diabetes

1. **Omega-3 Fatty Acids**: Found in high concentrations in Hilsa, Rohu, and Catla, these fatty acids help improve insulin sensitivity, reduce systemic inflammation, and lower the risk of heart disease, which is a common complication of diabetes.
2. **High-Quality Protein**: All these fish are excellent sources of protein, which is essential for repairing body tissues, maintaining muscle mass, and regulating blood sugar levels by slowing down the digestion and absorption of carbohydrates.
3. **Essential Vitamins and Minerals**: Vitamins like B12 and D, and minerals such as calcium, iron, and zinc, found in these fish, support overall metabolic health, enhance immune function, and contribute to the regulation of blood glucose levels.

Practical Tips for Incorporating Fish into a Diabetic Diet

- **Cooking Methods**: Opt for grilling, baking, steaming, or poaching fish to retain their nutritional benefits without adding unhealthy fats. Avoid frying, as it increases calorie and unhealthy fat intake.
- **Portion Control**: Consuming appropriate portion sizes ensures balanced calorie intake and maximizes health benefits.

- **Balanced Diet**: Pair fish with a variety of vegetables, whole grains, and healthy fats to create a well-rounded diet that supports overall metabolic health and blood sugar management.

Several types of fish are known to have beneficial effects for people with diabetes due to their high content of omega-3 fatty acids, high-quality protein, and low carbohydrate content. However, while no fish is specifically labeled as "anti-diabetic," certain fish can help manage blood sugar levels and improve overall metabolic health, which can be beneficial for individuals with diabetes. Here are some key fish that are particularly beneficial for people with diabetes:

1. Salmon (Salmo salar)
- **Nutritional Profile**: Rich in omega-3 fatty acids (EPA and DHA), high-quality protein, vitamin D, and selenium.
- **Benefits**: Omega-3s can improve insulin sensitivity, reduce inflammation, and lower the risk of heart disease, which is particularly important for people with diabetes.

2. Mackerel (Scomber scombrus)
- **Nutritional Profile**: High in omega-3 fatty acids, protein, vitamin B12, and selenium.
- **Benefits**: Omega-3s in mackerel can help reduce inflammation and improve cardiovascular health, which are common concerns for diabetic individuals.

3. Sardines (Sardinella spp.)
- **Nutritional Profile**: Rich in omega-3 fatty acids, vitamin D, calcium (when eaten with bones), and protein.
- **Benefits**: The high omega-3 content helps improve lipid profiles and reduce inflammation, which can enhance overall metabolic health.

4. Trout (Oncorhynchus mykiss)
- **Nutritional Profile**: High in omega-3 fatty acids, protein, vitamin B6, and vitamin B12.
- **Benefits**: Helps in managing blood sugar levels and improving insulin sensitivity.

5. Herring (Clupea harengus)
- **Nutritional Profile**: High in omega-3 fatty acids, vitamin D, and protein.
- **Benefits**: Omega-3 fatty acids in herring can improve heart health and reduce inflammation, which is beneficial for diabetic patients.

187

6. Tuna (Thunnus spp.)
- **Nutritional Profile**: High in protein, omega-3 fatty acids, and vitamin D.
- **Benefits**: Helps in reducing inflammation and improving cardiovascular health, which is essential for managing diabetes.

Mechanisms of Anti-Diabetic Effects

1. **Omega-3 Fatty Acids**:
   - **Insulin Sensitivity**: Omega-3 fatty acids can improve insulin sensitivity, helping to regulate blood glucose levels.
   - **Anti-Inflammatory**: They reduce inflammation, which is often elevated in diabetic individuals and is associated with insulin resistance.
   - **Cardiovascular Health**: Reducing triglycerides and improving cholesterol levels, which is crucial since diabetes significantly increases the risk of cardiovascular disease.
2. **High-Quality Protein**:
   - **Blood Sugar Regulation**: Protein helps regulate blood sugar levels by slowing down the absorption of carbohydrates and reducing spikes in blood glucose.
   - **Satiety**: Protein increases satiety, helping to control appetite and reduce overeating, which can be beneficial for weight management and blood sugar control.
3. **Low Carbohydrate Content**:
   - **Glycemic Control**: Fish is naturally low in carbohydrates, making it an excellent food choice for maintaining stable blood sugar levels.

Additional Recommendations
- **Preparation Methods**: To maximize health benefits, prepare fish using healthy methods such as grilling, baking, steaming, or poaching. Avoid frying, which adds unhealthy fats and calories.
- **Portion Control**: Maintain appropriate portion sizes to balance calorie intake and prevent excessive consumption of fats.
- **Balanced Diet**: Incorporate fish as part of a balanced diet that includes a variety of vegetables, whole grains, and healthy fats to support overall metabolic health.

Bangladeshi Fish and Psoriasis

Psoriasis is a chronic autoimmune condition characterized by the rapid growth of skin cells leading to scaling and inflammation. Diet, including the consumption of certain types of fish, can play a role in managing the symptoms of psoriasis due to their anti-inflammatory properties and high content of omega-3 fatty acids. In Bangladesh, several types of fish are beneficial for individuals with psoriasis:

1. Hilsa (Tenualosa ilisha)
- **Nutritional Profile**: High in omega-3 fatty acids, protein, and essential vitamins like vitamin D and B12.
- **Benefits**: Omega-3s help reduce inflammation and may alleviate the symptoms of psoriasis. Vitamin D is also known for its role in skin health.

2. Rohu (Labeo rohita)
- **Nutritional Profile**: Contains omega-3 and omega-6 fatty acids, high-quality protein, and essential minerals like zinc and selenium.
- **Benefits**: The anti-inflammatory properties of omega-3s and the immune-boosting effects of zinc and selenium can help manage psoriasis symptoms.

3. Catla (Catla catla)
- **Nutritional Profile**: Rich in protein, omega-3 fatty acids, and essential minerals such as phosphorus and calcium.
- **Benefits**: Omega-3s reduce inflammation and improve skin health, while protein supports overall health.

4. Tilapia (Oreochromis niloticus)
- **Nutritional Profile**: High in protein, moderate in omega-3 fatty acids, and contains vitamins and minerals essential for skin health.
- **Benefits**: Supports muscle health and skin repair, helping to manage the symptoms of psoriasis.

5. Pangasius (Pangasius pangasius)
- **Nutritional Profile**: High in protein and omega-3 fatty acids, low in saturated fats.
- **Benefits**: Provides essential nutrients for reducing inflammation and maintaining healthy skin.

Specific Benefits for Managing Psoriasis

1. **Omega-3 Fatty Acids**:

189

- o **Anti-Inflammatory Properties**: Omega-3s can help reduce inflammation, which is a key component of psoriasis.
- o **Skin Health**: Omega-3s support the maintenance of healthy skin and may reduce the severity of psoriasis flare-ups.

2. **High-Quality Protein:**
   - o **Skin Repair**: Protein is essential for the repair and regeneration of skin cells, which can help manage psoriasis symptoms.
   - o **Overall Health**: Protein supports the body's overall health, aiding in the management of autoimmune conditions like psoriasis.

3. **Vitamins and Minerals:**
   - o **Vitamin D**: Found in Hilsa, it helps regulate skin cell growth and can reduce the severity of psoriasis.
   - o **Zinc and Selenium**: Present in Rohu and Catla, these minerals boost immune function and have anti-inflammatory properties that benefit skin health.

Practical Tips for Incorporating Fish into a Psoriasis-Friendly Diet

- **Healthy Cooking Methods**: Choose grilling, baking, steaming, or poaching to preserve the fish's nutrients and avoid added unhealthy fats.
- **Balanced Diet**: Combine fish with a variety of vegetables, whole grains, and healthy fats to create a diet that supports overall health and reduces inflammation.
- **Regular Consumption**: Include fish in your diet regularly to benefit from their anti-inflammatory properties and essential nutrients.

Anti-Aging and fish

Here are some fish, including those commonly found in Bangladesh, that are beneficial for anti-aging due to their high nutritional content:

1. Salmon (Salmo salar)
- **Benefits**: Rich in omega-3 fatty acids, which help reduce inflammation, maintain skin elasticity, and promote heart health.

2. Hilsa (Tenualosa ilisha)
- **Benefits**: High in omega-3s and vitamin D, supporting skin health and reducing oxidative stress.

3. Mackerel (Scomber scombrus)
- **Benefits**: Packed with omega-3 fatty acids and antioxidants, which protect against cellular damage and promote youthful skin.

4. Rohu (Labeo rohita)
- **Benefits**: Contains high-quality protein and essential amino acids that support skin repair and regeneration.

5. Catla (Catla catla)
- **Benefits**: Rich in omega-3s and vitamins, aiding in maintaining skin health and reducing signs of aging.

6. Sardines (Sardinella longiceps)
- **Benefits**: High in omega-3s and vitamin B12, supporting brain health and reducing the risk of age-related cognitive decline.

7. Tuna (Thunnus spp.)
- **Benefits**: Provides high-quality protein and omega-3s, contributing to overall health and skin vitality.

8. Tilapia (Oreochromis niloticus)
- **Benefits**: A good source of protein, promoting healthy skin and muscle maintenance.

Nutritional Components Beneficial for Anti-Aging
- **Omega-3 Fatty Acids**: Reduce inflammation, improve skin hydration, and support heart health.
- **Antioxidants**: Protect against oxidative stress, which contributes to aging.
- **High-Quality Protein**: Supports skin repair and maintenance of muscle mass.
- **Vitamins (D, B12, E)**: Essential for skin health, cognitive function, and overall vitality.

Practical Tips
- **Cooking Methods**: Opt for grilling, baking, or steaming to preserve nutrients.
- **Regular Consumption**: Include fish in your diet regularly to maximize health benefits.

Incorporating these fish into a balanced diet can help promote healthier, more youthful skin and overall well-being.

Blood Group Compatibility with Bangladeshi Fish

Here's a general guide on which Bangladeshi fish may be suited for different human blood groups based on common dietary preferences:

1. **Blood Group A**

    o **Recommended Fish:**
- **Hilsa (Tenualosa ilisha)**
- **Rohu (Labeo rohita)**

    o **Notes:** Prefer plant-based diets; lean fish is suitable.

2. **Blood Group B**
    o **Recommended Fish:**
- **Catfish (Ictalurus spp.)**
- **Mackerel (Rastrelliger kanagurta)**

    o **Notes:** Can handle a variety of foods, including some fatty fish.

3. **Blood Group AB**
    o **Recommended Fish:**
- **Salmon (if available)**
- **Pomfret (Parastromateus niger)**

    o **Notes:** Can digest a wide range of foods, including both lean and fatty fish.

4. **Blood Group O**
    o **Recommended Fish:**
- **Tuna (Thunnus spp.)**
- **Hilsa (Tenualosa ilisha)**

Bangladeshi Fish with Low Glycemic Index

Fish generally have a low glycemic index (GI) because they contain minimal carbohydrates. However, here are some Bangladeshi fish known for their nutrient profiles, which are low in GI:

1. **Hilsa (Tenualosa ilisha)**
2. **Rohu (Labeo rohita)**
3. **Catfish (Ictalurus spp.)**
4. **Mackerel (Rastrelliger kanagurta)**
5. **Pomfret (Parastromateus niger)**
   Bangladeshi Fish that May Help Prevent Heart Attacks
   These fish are good choices for maintaining stable blood sugar levels. For specific dietary concerns, consult a healthcare professional.

Here are some Bangladeshi fish known to be beneficial for heart health:

1. Hilsa (Tenualosa ilisha)

- o Rich in omega-3 fatty acids, which can reduce inflammation and improve heart health.
2. **Rohu (Labeo rohita)**
   - o Contains healthy fats that support cardiovascular health.
3. **Mackerel (Rastrelliger kanagurta)**
   - o High in omega-3s, promoting better cholesterol levels.
4. **Catfish (Ictalurus spp.)**
   - o Provides lean protein and essential nutrients beneficial for heart health.
5. **Pomfret (Parastromateus niger)**
   - o Good source of omega-3 fatty acids and low in saturated fat.

Immune Booster Fishes

Fish can be an excellent source of nutrients that support the immune system. Here are some Bangladeshi fish, both big and small, that are good for boosting the immune system:

Small Fish

1. **Mola (Amblypharyngodon mola)**
   - o **Nutritional Benefits**: Rich in vitamin A and calcium, essential for immune function.
   - o **Omega-3 Fatty Acids**: Supports immune health and reduces inflammation.
2. **Tangra (Mystus tengara)**
   - o **Nutritional Benefits**: Good source of protein and essential minerals like zinc, which plays a critical role in immune function.
   - o **B Vitamins**: Supports overall immune health.
3. **Puti (Puntius sophore)**
   - o **Nutritional Benefits**: High in protein and micronutrients such as iron and zinc.
   - o **Antioxidants**: Contains vitamins and minerals that help protect cells from oxidative stress.

Big Fish

1. **Hilsa (Tenualosa ilisha)**
   - o **Nutritional Benefits**: High in omega-3 fatty acids, which enhance immune function and reduce inflammation.

193

    o   **Vitamin D**: Important for immune regulation and response.
2. **Rohu (Labeo rohita)**
    o   **Nutritional Benefits**: Rich in protein, omega-3 fatty acids, and vitamins like B12 and D.
    o   **Micronutrients**: Contains selenium, which is crucial for a healthy immune system.
3. **Catla (Catla catla)**
    o   **Nutritional Benefits**: Provides high-quality protein and essential fatty acids.
    o   **Vitamins and Minerals**: Contains vitamins A, D, and B-complex, along with minerals like iron and zinc.

Additional Recommendations

- **Variety**: Consuming a variety of fish ensures a broad spectrum of nutrients.
- **Preparation**: Cooking methods such as steaming, grilling, or baking help preserve the nutrients in fish.
- **Balanced Diet**: Incorporate fish as part of a balanced diet with vegetables, fruits, and whole grains to support overall immune health.

Fish Combinations to Avoid
1. **Tuna and Mackerel**
    o   Both can contain high levels of mercury.
2. **Fish with High Histamine (e.g., Sardines, Anchovies)**
    o   Avoid combining with other high-histamine foods to prevent reactions.
3. **Raw Fish and Shellfish**
    o   Consuming raw fish with raw shellfish can increase the risk of foodborne illness.
4. **Smoked Fish with Certain Cheeses**
    o   The combination can lead to increased histamine levels, causing allergic reactions.
5. **Different Types of Fish**
    o   Mixing fatty and lean fish can alter cooking times and textures, leading to uneven cooking.

General Tips
- **Mercury Levels**: Be cautious about combining fish with high mercury content.
- **Dietary Restrictions**: Consider individual allergies and intolerances when combining seafood.

Mercury

Yes, freshwater fish in Bangladesh can contain mercury due to various environmental factors. Here are some key points:

Sources of Mercury in Freshwater Fish

1. **Industrial Pollution**: Runoff from factories can lead to mercury entering water bodies.
2. **Agricultural Runoff**: Pesticides and fertilizers can contribute to water contamination.
3. **Sediment Resuspension**: Mercury present in sediments can be released into the water.

Freshwater Fish in Bangladesh with Potential Mercury Exposure
1. **Rohu (Labeo rohita)**
2. **Catfish (Ictalurus spp.)**
3. **Hilsa (Tenualosa ilisha)** (when found in freshwater)
4. **Mrigal (Cirrhinus mrigala)**

Health Implications
- **Bioaccumulation**: Mercury accumulates in fish tissues over time, posing risks to consumers.
- **Health Risks**: Consumption of contaminated fish can lead to neurological and developmental issues.

Effects of Mercury Consumption through Fish

1. **Neurological Damage**
   o   Mercury can affect the brain, leading to cognitive deficits, memory loss, and developmental issues, particularly in children.
2. **Cardiovascular Issues**
   o   Mercury exposure may increase the risk of heart disease and hypertension.
3. **Kidney Damage**
   o   High levels of mercury can impair kidney function, potentially leading to kidney disease.
4. **Immune System Suppression**

- o Mercury can weaken the immune response, making the body more susceptible to infections.
5. **Reproductive and Developmental Effects**
   - o Exposure during pregnancy can lead to developmental delays and birth defects in infants.
6. **Gastrointestinal Symptoms**
   - o Consumption of mercury-laden fish can cause nausea, vomiting, and abdominal pain.

Mercury Levels in Fish by Region

1. North America
- **Species**: Tuna, Swordfish, Shark
- **Mercury Levels**: 0.3 - 1.0 ppm (parts per million)

2. Europe
- **Species**: Pike, Haddock
- **Mercury Levels**: 0.1 - 0.5 ppm

3. Asia (including Bangladesh)
- **Species**: Hilsa, Catfish
- **Mercury Levels**: 0.2 - 0.7 ppm

4. South America
- **Species**: Tarpon, Tuna
- **Mercury Levels**: 0.3 - 1.2 ppm

General Trends
- **High-Mercury Fish**: Shark, Swordfish, King Mackerel, and some Tuna.
- **Low-Mercury Fish**: Salmon, Sardines, and Catfish.

Types of Mercury Found in Fish by Region

1. **Methylmercury**
   - o **Region**: Worldwide
   - o **Description**: The most toxic form of mercury, primarily found in fish due to bioaccumulation in aquatic food chains.
2. **Elemental Mercury**
   - o **Region**: Commonly in industrial areas

- o **Description**: Released from industrial processes; can convert to methylmercury in aquatic environments.
3. **Inorganic Mercury**
    - o **Region**: Various freshwater and coastal areas
    - o **Description**: Comes from mining and industrial runoff; less commonly found in fish compared to methylmercury.

Regional Highlights
- **North America**
    - o **Common Species**: Tuna, Swordfish
    - o **Mercury Type**: Primarily methylmercury.
- **Europe**
    - o **Common Species**: Pike, Haddock
    - o **Mercury Type**: Mainly methylmercury, with some presence of inorganic mercury.
- **Asia (including Bangladesh)**
    - o **Common Species**: Hilsa, Catfish
    - o **Mercury Type**: Predominantly methylmercury due to industrial pollution and fish farming practices.
- **South America**
    - o **Common Species**: Tarpon, Tuna
    - o **Mercury Type**: Mainly methylmercury, especially in regions with gold mining.

Conclusion

Methylmercury is the primary concern for fish consumption globally, resulting from environmental contamination and bioaccumulation in aquatic ecosystems.

References/Sources

The information about mercury in freshwater fish in Bangladesh can be found in various studies and reports from the following sources:

1. **World Health Organization (WHO)**: Provides guidelines on mercury exposure and health effects.
2. **Food and Agriculture Organization (FAO)**: Offers insights into fisheries and aquaculture in developing countries.
3. **Local Environmental Studies**: Research articles and journals focusing on environmental pollution in Bangladesh, such as those found in academic databases like Google Scholar.
4. **Bangladesh's Department of Fisheries**: Reports on fish health and contamination levels.

Here are some authoritative sources you can refer to for detailed nutritional information on Bagarius species and similar fish:

1. USDA FoodData Central
   - Provides comprehensive nutritional data for a wide range of foods, including fish. You can search for specific species.
   - FoodData Central
2. NutritionData (Self.com)
   - Offers detailed nutrition profiles for many foods, including fish.
   - NutritionData
3. Food and Agriculture Organization (FAO)
   - Provides reports and databases on fish species, including their nutritional content.
   - FAO Fisheries & Aquaculture
4. Research Articles and Journals
   - Search for articles on platforms like Google Scholar or PubMed. Look for studies focusing on the nutritional analysis of specific fish species.
   - Google Scholar
5. FishBase
   - A comprehensive database on fish species that includes biological and nutritional information.
   - FishBase
6. Peer-Reviewed Journals
   - Journals such as "Journal of Fish Biology" and "Aquaculture" often publish studies on fish nutrition and health.

Suggested Research Strategies
   - **Use Specific Keywords**: When searching, use terms like "nutritional profile of Bagarius species" or "nutritional analysis of freshwater fish".

- **Look for Regional Studies**: Some studies focus on fish species common in specific regions, which may provide more accurate data.

Example References

1. **Bachman, R. (1993)**. Nutritional profiles of various fish species. *Journal of Aquatic Food Product Technology*.
2. **FAO. (2018)**. Fishery and aquaculture statistics. *FAO Yearbook*.
3. **Zhou, X., & Pan, Y. (2016)**. Nutritional value of freshwater fish. *Aquaculture Nutrition*.

By consulting these sources, you can obtain the most accurate and detailed nutritional information for Bagarius and other fish species.